A CLASSIC APPROACH TO

MAKE-UP

FOR FASHION, FILM & THEATRE

BY MARK TRAYNOR

Project Editor: Joan Leahey

Acknowledgements

I would like to thank my
friends and great make-up artists
Donald Lee
Edward Jackson
Stan Place
Sherne
and
Randy Mercer
for their helpful suggestions

Photography
by
Don Manza
Mark Traynor
Robert Jordon

Table of Contents

Chapter 6: Face-Lifting Techniques for the Make-up Artist

Section 2—Fashion, Film and Theatre

Chapter 7: Choosing Make-up for Various Media

About the Author

Mark Traynor is not one to rest on his laurels. He is a constant innovator, a professional, and world famous in his chosen field. As an imaginative make-up artist, hair stylist, photographer and beauty consultant to many of the world's most beautiful women, he is the foremost proponent of the "total look" in beauty.

Mark Traynor's entire career has been devoted to the glorification and enhancement of feminine beauty. He has been professionally involved with and consulted by such stars as Ginger Rogers, Marilyn Monroe, Lauren Hutton, Cheryl Tiegs, Jennifer O'Neill, model Iman, Barbara Walters, Joan Rivers, Wilhelmina, to name just a few.

Aside from professional beauties, Mr. Traynor realizes the world is filled with women whose ultimate beauty potential has never been tapped, and it is these women who can benefit most from the Traynor Method of Beauty.

A true artist, Mark Traynor uses as his canvas the female face. He has done hundreds of magazine covers, adorned models for even more fashion layouts, appeared on Johnny Carson, Merv Griffin, Mike Douglas and David Frost Shows dozens of times, and he is responsible for the beautiful appearance of hundreds of models on TV commercials. He also has created the make-up for The Miss New York State, Miss World and Miss Universe pageant contestants.

Many of Mark Traynor's innovations have been widely copied; such as face-painting, multi-colored hair, jeweled wigs; and for men—wigs, false brows and beards, all that slip on instantly. His now famous Temporary Face Lift and his Isometric Beauty Band have revolutionized the beauty world. With them, a woman can literally make time appear to stand still.

He is the author of "The New Beauty," "Sculpture Styling," "The Professional Make-up Artist Guide" and "The Mark Traynor Beauty Book" from Doubleday.

Mark Traynor Cosmetics, Inc., developed in 1970, features a product line now sold at more than 1,500 beauty salons and cosmetic boutiques throughout the United States and Canada.

Mark Traynor has also been the Make-up Director for the Wilfred Academy schools since 1966. Many of the famous make-up artists for film, fashion and television have originally studied make-up in the Wilfred Academy.

Introduction to Make-up

Here is a book designed for the serious make-up student. Written in simple language, it details various forms of make-up from simple daytime make-up through the specialized techniques for Fashion Photography, Television and Theatre. It fills the gap between the simplistic books on corrective and fashion make-up and the more formal books on theatrical make-up which may be difficult for the beginning student to understand. Every step of each type of make-up is graphically detailed in illustrations and text. This is the ideal book for the make-up student whether he or she plans a career as a make-up artist, a model or as an actor or actress.

HISTORY OF MAKE-UP

For the uninitiated, professional make-up is a great mystery. Yet taught in a step-by-step manner the mystery unfolds and becomes relatively simple. It is important to understand the background of the use of cosmetics throughout the history of mankind.

Cosmetics in one form or another have been used to adorn the human body since mankind learned to walk erect. In certain periods both men and women used cosmetics while in other periods of history only one of the sexes availed themselves of cosmetics for adornment. The theatre is the only area in which cosmetics have always been used. This use stems from the need to accentuate a character's features so they project into the audience or the need to change someone's features to create a different character.

During the Victorian period the use of cosmetics was frowned upon and only actresses and so called "ladies of the evening" used them. It was not until the advent of silent movies that cosmetics came back into popular use. How this came about is interesting to contemplate.

The first movies were silent and shot in black and white film. The strong lights had a tendency to wash out the features so that make-up was necessary to define the features. As this was a totally new medium, there were no specialized make-up artists, and actors and actresses were expected to apply their own make-up. Since almost all of the performers were trained for theatre they used the very same theatre make-up techniques when applying make-up for the screen. They did not take into consideration the closeups and the searching eye of the camera. The outcome as can be seen in early films is the heavily outlined eyes, the rouged cheeks and seemingly black lipsticks. This look of course was nothing more than the highly accentuating theatre make-up which, when filmed, caused deep reds to turn black and outlined eyes to look completely unnatural. Of course as things progressed make-up became more sophisticated.

Women everywhere took the screen heroines to their hearts and tried to emulate them. Famous screen stars such as Mary Pickford, Clara Bow, and Pola Negri, to name but a few, started the fads of the cupid's bow lipshape, the rouged cheek and the thin arched brow. And so we entered an era which extends into today where the use of cosmetics by women is as normal as brushing the teeth or having the hair styled.

The evolution of contemporary make-up

Make-up fashions change as often as hairstyles do and in fact sometimes more often. It may be a change in the technique of application or it may be in the colors used. From the 1930's to the 1950's make-up was applied in more or less a basic manner—fluid make-up to smooth out the complexion, cream rouge for cheek color, powder for a matte finish, a color eye-shadow to complement the eye color, mascara, eye-liner, brow pencil and lip color. This was standard and varied only in the colors used and in the application. It was towards the end of the 1950's that make-up artists who worked in theatre, film and television started to bring their expertise and knowledge to cosmetic manufacturers and fashion magazines. Thus techniques heretofore used solely for theatrical effects became a standard part of everyday make-up.

The classic techniques

The classic standards of beauty were set down thousands of years ago by Grecian artists. It is they who set forth the oval-shaped face as the most beautiful and set down facial proportions that they deemed the most perfect. It is to these ideals that we still cling. The professional make-up artist, adapting make-up application techniques from the theatre, attempts to bring out each individual client's beauty, hide her flaws, and in general create a look of classic beauty.

THE CONTEMPORARY LOOK

In a more up-to-date approach to make-up, the make-up artist does not slavishly cling to the ideal of creating a classic look. Rather, the artist adds these standards to the more modern method of treating each and every client as an individual and attempts to create a look of beauty within their own personality type.

The fashion influence

A new make-up look is created in many ways. Eye-liner, for example, was out of fashion for many years and yet returned when designers brought Indian Saris into the fashion picture. Models used black Kohl to surround their eyes in the Indian manner and a new eye make-up look was established. Sometimes a clothing designer will call in a hairstylist and make-up artist to create a new look on his models that will enhance and coordinate with his new creations. Colors will be picked from the collection, fashion magazines will take note of the new look and cosmetic manufacturers will begin to produce new shades and new cosmetics as a follow through. Voila, a new make-up fashion is announced. It might also be a look worn by a film or television star that catches the public's fancy, or a look established by a famous model. Think back to the Farrah Fawcett hairdo, the Egyptian eye make-up worn by Elizabeth Taylor as Cleopatra or the funny little painted eyelashes of Twiggy, the English model of the 60's. The public loves to follow and pick up on anything new, exciting and different.

The chiaroscuro approach

Chiaroscuro in art is the use of light and shadow to create a sculptured effect. Using this principle the make-up artist can appear to change the shape of the face, slenderize a nose or contour a cheek. Using a minimal amount of color and utilizing mostly earth tones that range from ivory to dark brown, the artist can create many illusions whether the desired effect is to beautify a client for a gala evening or create an aged character make-up for the stage. In the late 1950's and early 1960's make-up artists started adapting these principles and techniques to everyday make-up. The contouring and sculpturing so useful in black and white photography became the regular make-up of the fashion conscious woman, sometimes to good effect and sometimes very overdone. Still, it brought a new professionalism to the application of make-up. The artist uses the Chiaroscuro technique in almost every media where make-up is applied but most successfully on stage where the actor or actress is viewed from a distance allowing an illusion to approach reality.

BEGIN AT THE BEGINNING

Let us start on our career as a make-up artist with the realization that there is no such thing as too much knowledge. Many artists feel that they only want to be a fashion make-up artist in a salon, make-up studio or school. What a grievous mistake it is to limit one's knowledge. You never know what type of make-up you may be required to do or down which road your career may lead you. You may work in a beauty salon as a make-up artist, as a consultant at a cosmetic counter, or for a cosmetic company as a technical consultant in charge of helping to create a new cosmetic line. You may want to teach make-up in a beauty school, train actors and actresses in theatrical make-up techniques or work in television or film. Perhaps you would like to specialize as a photographer's make-up artist or just make brides beautiful for their wedding day. The list is endless.

What you must keep in mind is that make-up for all media is interrelated. That is why it is essential to start at the beginning, so that in the final analysis you will thoroughly understand all there is to know about the art of the professional make-up artist. This book attempts to simplify even the most intricate techniques so that your career will be off to a flying start.

Section 1

A Classic Approach to Make-up

Chapter 1

Facial Anatomy

Though it is not necessary to have a highly technical knowledge of anatomy, it is important to understand the basic structure of the face so you can create anything from a more beautifully shaped face to a new character for an actor or actress.

THE MUSCLES OF THE FACE

The muscles of the face control facial expression and work by contraction. The skin forms the expression and is wrinkled at right angles to the pull of the muscle. Knowing the muscles of the face and their placement will aid the make-up artist when the depiction of an aged character is called for.

The muscles of the face that are important in relation to make-up are:

Frontalis—This muscle animates the forehead and brow. (No. 1)

Orbicularis Oculi—This muscle completely surrounds the eye and controls the opening, closing and blinking of the eyes. (No. 2)

Zygomaticus—This muscle aids in facial expressions such as smiling and laughing. (No. 3)

Orbicularis Oris—This muscle completely surrounds the lips and draws the lips together for variety of facial expressions such as pouting or whistling. (No. 4)

Buccinator—This muscle draws back the inner angle of the mouth and flattens the lips against the teeth. (No. 5)

Corrugator—This draws the inner angle of the eyebrow in and down to cause frowning. (No. 6)

Temporalis and Masseter—These two muscles coordinate in the raising of the jawbone (mandible) for the chewing process. (No. 7 and No. 8)

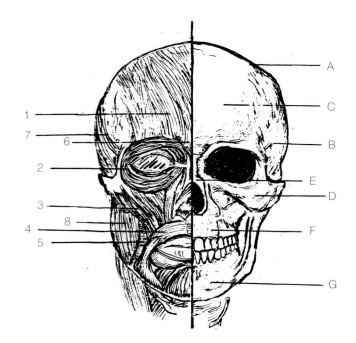

THE BONES OF THE FACE AND HEAD

Understanding the placement and shape of the bones of the face and skull will assist you in techniques such as the proper sculpturing of the cheek bones, contouring the eyes, aging of an actor and changing an Occidental into an Oriental. Indeed, these are many of the effects that you may be called upon to create whether you work as a make-up artist at a cosmetic counter or in a film studio.

The bones of the head, or skull, are held together by immovable joints, with the exception of the lower jaw. Basically there are two groups of bones: The bones of the head, or cranium, which protect the brain, and the bones of the face, which are of more immediate concern to the make-up artist. Refer to the illustration above for exact location of the bones that follow.

The bones of the cranium are:

> **Occipital Bone**—This forms the back and base of the cranium. It is to its under-surface that the muscles of the neck are connected. The spinal cord connects with the brain through the center of this undersurface. (Not seen on illustration)

> **Two Parietal Bones**—These are on either side of the cranium and cover the top of the skull. (Ltr. A)

> **Two Temporal Bones**—These form the lower part of the sides of the cranium. (Ltr. B)

> **Frontal Bone**—This is the front of the cranium, including what we call the forehead and brow bone. (Ltr. C)

The bones of the face are:

Two Zygomatic Bones—They form the cheek bone prominence, the zygomatic arch on either side of the face and part of the eye sockets. The temporal muscle passes beneath this arch. (Ltr. D)

Two Nasal Bones—These form the bridge or upper part of the nose. (Ltr. E)

Two Maxilla Bones—These form the upper jaw and part of the eye sockets. (Ltr. F)

Mandible Bone—This forms the lower jaw and chin, and connects beneath the zygomatic arches in front of the ears. (Ltr. G)

Study those around you and notice how the shape and size of the head and the facial structure varies from person to person. Look at the illustration of the skull and then feel and probe for the shape and placement of the bones of your own face. You can easily see why a prominent zygomatic arch will create well defined cheek bones and why a dominant frontal bone that forms a strong protective arch over the eyes will make for deep-set eyes. A working knowledge of the facial bones is indeed important to the make-up artist.

FACIAL SHAPES

Classically, the oval-shaped face is considered the ideal. Using the oval as a basis of comparison enables you to most easily recognize deviations from this shape. In cases where there is a desire to restructure or somewhat alter a feature or facial contour, the use of cleverly applied make-up will always help achieve this end. More recently, the rule to ovalize the facial shape does not have the significance it once had. The contemporary practice is to create a more or less individual "look" for each woman within a framework of their own features, personality and lifestyle. Although this is a fact of modern make-up, recognition of the various facial shapes and structures is the beginning of an approach to the problems of adjusting and placing into balance that which does not create a harmonious picture.

There are basically eight facial shapes which you should learn to recognize:

1. **The Oval:** In this facial shape, the temple and forehead are the widest area, tapering down to a curved chin. This is considered the most perfect facial shape because of its balance and overall look of symmetry.

2. **The Round:** Just as its name implies, this face is widest at the cheek bone area and is usually not much longer than it is wide. It has a softly rounded jawline, short chin, and a rounded hairline over a rather full forehead.

3. **The Square:** Starting from a straight hairline down to a square chin, this face has an angular jawline and not particularly prominent cheek bones. The lines of this face are straight and angular.

4. **The Oblong:** This face could also be described as rectangular since it is long and narrow. The cheeks are often hollowed under prominent cheek bones, and it is usually typified by an overly long, angular chin and/or a high forehead.

5. **The Triangle:** Like a pyramid, this face is widest at its base or jawline, tapering up to slightly narrower cheeks, and reaching its apex at a narrow forehead.

6. **The Inverted Triangle:** This facial shape has width at the temple and forehead area, tapering down to a narrow chin.

7. **The Heart Shape:** This face has a small, pointed chin, a narrow jawline, soft rather than angular contours, width at the cheek bone area and slightly less width at the forehead.

8. **The Diamond Shape:** This shape is somewhat similar to the heart-shaped face except that the forehead is narrower and the face more angular. The measurements of the jaw and hairline are approximately the same.

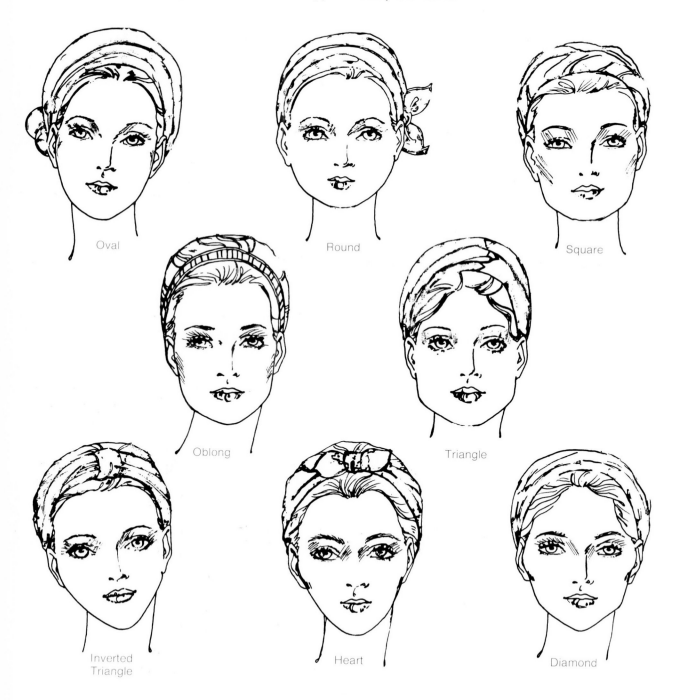

Oval

Round

Square

Oblong

Triangle

Inverted Triangle

Heart

Diamond

Facial shape, although still vitally important, is no longer the sole criterion upon which a successful make-up is executed. Other facial aspects must now be considered in order for the make-up artist to develop a total concept of the task ahead of him.

1. **Bone structure**—This is the basic foundation upon which your make-up must be constructed. It determines the planes and shadows which can be either heightened or diminished to achieve the desired effect.

2. **Skin texture**—Just as a painter determines the type of medium he will use by the texture of the canvas he has chosen, so you must choose the correct type of make-up for the texture of your client's skin.

3. **Features**—The size, shape and placement of the client's features must be evaluated in order to create the most attractive effect possible.

   It is important for you to be able to judge these essential factors at a glance.

FACIAL PROPORTIONS

As we utilize the oval-shaped face as a standard to judge the attractiveness of the facial contours, so we must have some standard by which to judge the proper proportions of the features. As a standard, we use the accepted classical measurements by which to judge the correct placement and balance of the features.

Judging the general balance of the face

Lengthwise, the face is divided horizontally into three equal sections:

1. From the center hairline to the lowest part of the inner portion of the eyebrows.

2. From the brow to the base of the nose.

3. From the base of the nose to the bottom of the chin.

If these sections are equal, the face may be considered to be in proper proportion lengthwise.

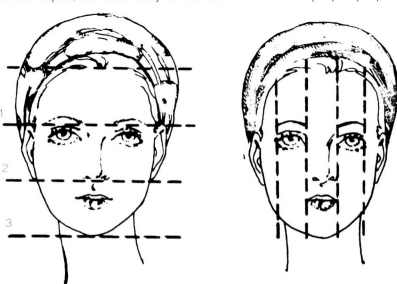

Across, the face can be divided vertically into three sections using the placement of the eyes as a guide. Proportionately, the space between the eyes should equal the width of one eye. Therefore, if the width of both eyes is the same and the space between the eyes equals the width of one eye, there is a correct balance.

Judging placement and proportions of lips

The proper placement and proportions of the lips can be judged by dividing the lower facial area into three sections as follows:

1. One third from the base of the nose to the center of the lips.

2. Two thirds from the center of the lips to the base of the chin.

3. The width of the mouth may be approximately the distance between the irises of the eyes.

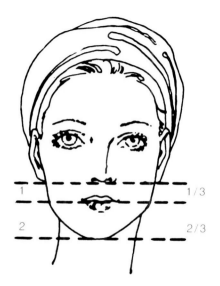 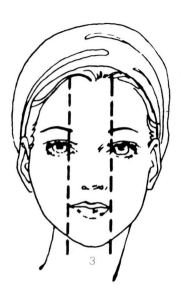

Profiles

Though much can be done through illusion to alter and affect the shape of the face and its features from front view, very little can be done with regular make-up to alter the profile. Generally profiles can be affected with the proper hairdress.

1. **Straight Profile:** This profile is considered ideal.

2. **Convex Profile:** This profile may have a slanted forehead and a small or slightly receding chin.

3. **Concave Profile:** This profile may feature a rounded or prominent forehead and an exaggerated or jutting chin line.

Once you are able to judge your client's general facial contours and proportions, you can proceed to plan a harmonious and balanced make-up. Of course, through experience, you will learn to perceive all of this with just a moment's study of the face and features.

Judging eye placement

The eyes are the most expressive of features and the focal point of the face. Special care must therefore be taken when applying eye make-up to emphasize their dramatic qualities while maintaining the over-all balance of the face. Because they draw more attention than any other feature, the eyes must be made-up with extreme care. Any flaw will attract immediate attention and thus diminish the beauty of an otherwise perfect make-up.

The eye is basically divided into three areas; the eyelid, the depth area, and the brow bone. The ideally proportioned upper eye area would be divided as follows: One third from the base of the lashes to the crease line, and two thirds from the crease line to the eyebrow. There are, of course, many variations ranging from the very heavy-lidded eye to the flat-lidded eye of the Oriental.

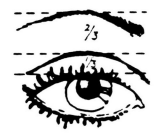

The upper eye area
proportions

The well-spaced eye has the width of one eye between the eyes.

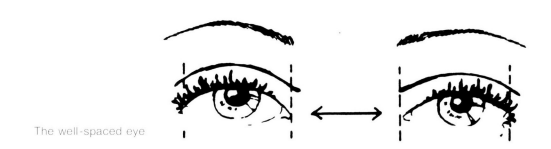

The well-spaced eye

Until you learn to judge eye placement by simple recognition, you can measure the eyes with the liner brush. First measure the length of one eye and place that length of brush between the eyes from one inner corner to the other.

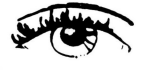
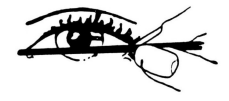

Measuring the eye with
a brush

To be more exacting, a pair of calipers may be used. This will add a touch of professionalism. An inexpensive pair of calipers can be obtained at an art-supply store or any shop selling drafting materials. First, place the calipers carefully against one eye, measuring its width. Keeping the calipers at the measurement, place the points of the calipers between the eyes from inner corner to inner corner (near the tear ducts.) Be very careful while doing this.

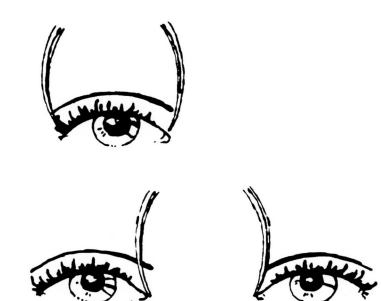

Using calipers to measure eye width

Using calipers to measure space between eyes

You can very simply judge now whether the eyes are evenly spaced or need correction.

Chapter 2

Lighting and Color

Good lighting is one of the most important requirements for doing really effective make-up. Ideally the lighting should approximate the light of the time of day and the place where the client will be. For instance, make-up seen outdoors on a sunny afternoon will appear radically different than it does in the dim light of a cocktail lounge in the evening. It is the difference in the lighting that changes the total aspect of the make-up. Understanding the differences in various lighting situations will greatly assist in the choice of cosmetic colors and their application.

LET'S TALK ABOUT LIGHTING

Daylight

Daylight is basically composed of four rays of the color spectrum—**Red, Yellow, Blue** and **Green.**

Red and yellow can be considered "warm colors" and blue and green are alluded to as "cool colors." On a sunny day there is more red and yellow to the color spectrum. An overcast day is a cooler day and there is more blue and green to the color spectrum.

Incandescent bulbs

Incandescent bulbs are the common type of household lights and emit only red and yellow rays. Candlelight, nightclub and restaurant lighting and tungsten lighting used by photographers can all be considered in the same general category. In varying degrees they all add a warm tone to the skin.

Incandescent lights, tungsten lights and spotlights will pick up and exaggerate any irridescence and shine in make-up.

11

Fluorescent bulbs

Fluorescent bulbs are the most common type of lighting used in offices and schools and emit only blue and green rays. Depending on the tint of their glass casing, they add a cool tone to colors and absorb reds. There are some fluorescent tubes on the market that simulate true daylight, and emit a warmer tone. These of course would be the preferred type of fluorescent tubing for make-up application.

Fluorescent lighting will absorb and flatten any irridescence in pearlized make-up just as it absorbs red.

REMEMBER—Incandescent bulbs add a WARM TONE to the skin. Most fluorescent bulbs add a COOL TONE to the skin absorbing reds and turning beige tones sallow.

Lighting for the make-up area

The ideal lighting for make-up is that which most closely approximates daylight and is composed of the four color rays: red, yellow, blue and green. Combining incandescent and fluorescent bulbs will give you the four color rays and will allow you to check the make-up under different lighting situations. To accomplish this, you might have incandescent bulbs surrounding the mirror on the top and sides, using 40 watt bulbs to a total of perhaps 500 to 700 watts. Then add a flourescent tube above them at the top of the mirror. There should be absolutely no lighting from under the mirror and no ceiling lights directly overhead to create unwanted facial shadows.

When doing the make-up keep both sets of lights on. To check the make-up for evening or photography leave on only the incandescent bulbs. To check the make-up for office or school lighting, leave on only the fluorescent bulbs. Whatever you do make sure that you have enough light to see well. This is most important if you are to do a perfect make-up.

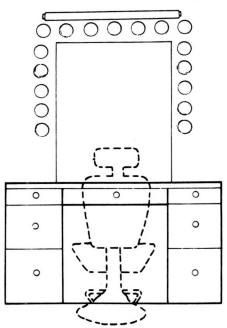

LET'S TALK ABOUT COLOR

A knowledge of color pigments is absolutely essential to the make-up artist. Just understanding the very basics will be of great help mixing and applying cosmetics.

Colors principles

There are three **primary** colors: RED, YELLOW and BLUE.

You obtain three **secondary** colors by mixing the primary colors together:

> Red and Yellow = ORANGE,
>
> Red and Blue = VIOLET,
>
> Blue and Yellow = GREEN.

The six **tertiary** or intermediate colors are:

> Red-orange
>
> Yellow-orange
>
> Yellow-green
>
> Blue-green
>
> Blue-violet
>
> Red-violet

Neutral colors are BLACK AND WHITE.

> Mix Black and White to make GREY
>
> Mix Black and Orange to make BROWN

So you see you can obtain practically any color you desire if you keep small containers of the following colors in cream form in your make-up kit: red, yellow, blue, white and black. These colors are known as **lining colors** and come in stick or cream form and are available wherever theatrical make-up is sold. The cream form is actually a better choice as it is more easily mixed together or added to other cosmetics.

Hue, intensity and value

The main characters of color are defined by the words **HUE**, **INTENSITY** and **VALUE**.

1. **Hue** is simply the name by which a color is known, such as, red, yellow, green, or blue.
2. **Intensity** denotes the relative brightness or dullness of a color. In other words a bright pure blue would be considered to be of high intensity. If grey were added to the blue, however, one would obtain a grey-blue which would be considered a blue of low intensity.
3. **Value** indicates the relative lightness or darkness of a color. An example would be adding white to red making pink. This would be considered a high value of red. By adding black to red one would come up with maroon. Maroon would be considered a low value of red.

Here are some further examples:

HUE	HIGH VALUE (add white)	LOW VALUE (add black)
Blue	Sky Blue	Indigo
Red	Pink	Maroon
Yellow	Ivory	Olive
Orange	Peach	Brown
Violet	Lilac	Purple
Green	Pale Green	Forest Green

Complementary colors

These colors are found opposite each other on an artist's color wheel. Examples would be blue and orange; yellow and violet; red and green. When used with discretion these combinations literally compliment each other in wardrobe and cosmetic use.

THE COLOR WHEEL

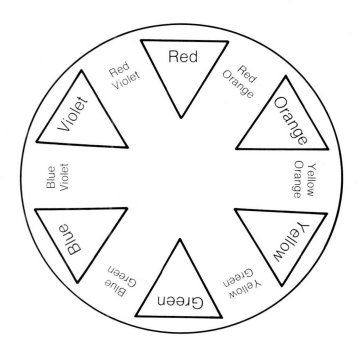

Chapter 3

Designing a Look

Before designing a make-up one must take many things into consideration. The facial shape, body structure, hairstyle, clothes and personality type are some of the major factors contributing to the final design of the make-up. The situation under which the make-up will be seen is also important. Is it for theatre and if so, is it a large or small theatre? Is it for television or film or to be photographed for print? Is the make-up a basic corrective one or is it to be a character make-up for the stage?

In most cases you will find that the application techniques for all media or situations are similar, with the changes occurring in the strength of the application and the colors used. The actual manner in which make-up is applied is the same in most cases since corrective make-up is based on the classic "Grecian Canons of Beauty," which are facial proportions set down by ancient Grecian artists as being ideal. To attain this ideal facial look we use the chiaroscuro approach of sculpturing the features and contouring the face through the use of highlights and shadows.

Let us start with creating a basic corrective make-up for everyday wear. The concept of designing a 'look' around the shape of the face is not of prime importance. The contemporary feeling in beauty is to build a theme that is individual; an overall picture that states the personality within the framework of fashion. The important thing is to create the total look of beauty coordinating the make-up with the hairstyle and clothing.

PERSONALITY

When designing a look, first determine the client's general personality. Is she sophisticated, tailored, or a romantic-feminine type? She may look high-fashion or fall into the category that most women do. That category is the woman who just wants to look prettier—to emphasize her good features, disguise her bad ones, and all with a minimum of effort.

The sophisticate or high fashion type is more interested in the latest fashion and is willing to spend extra time and effort to achieve unusual effects. New themes and colors and a more dramatic application of make-up may be used.

The **outdoor type** of woman requires extra attention to her skin-care program. A good make-up base, eye make-up, lipstick and blush will usually comprise her average make-up application.

The **tailored type** will want a no-nonsense approach to the make-up question. She will probably prefer a low key make-up that is fairly natural looking. A good basic make-up and skin-care program that suits her usual practical approach to things will find her most receptive.

The **feminine-romantic type** will love all things soft and pretty. Pastel colorings and subtle shadings and make-up suggestive of the glow of candlelight will turn romantic fantasies in the right direction. For the average woman, assuming there is one, you can do no wrong by making her as "pretty as a picture."

The **trendy type** is the opposite of the romantic. She likes to look individual and different. If it is "in" then it is "her," so long as it is different and definitely new. With it all, she likes to add her own particular touch to the finished product.

AGE GROUP

The second step in designing a look is to determine if the individual is a teenager, between the ages of twenty and forty or in her mature years. This must be considered, not only in terms of make-up and hairstyle but when choosing fashions as well. There is a blurring of lines in the last two decades and a tendency for the mature woman to strive for a younger look as well as a tendency for the teenager to look more mature than her years. The important thing is for a woman to look and feel well for her years.

For the teenager, the desired effect is that of naturalness and a light hand should be used in applying make-up. Use a water base make-up foundation when necessary. If the skin is flawless, a little moisturizer and a dusting of powder may be all that is needed as a base. Eye make-up, blush and lip color should all be applied lightly with a general effect of cleanliness and simplicity.

From the young twenties through the forties a full complement of cosmetics may be used to advantage in enhancing the woman's appearance.

The mature woman should use cosmetics with discretion. If the skin is lined with wrinkles a heavy application of make-up will make the mature woman look her years and more. Care should be taken to avoid excessive use of blush and eye-liner and the heavily powdered look.

OCCASION

The third step for designing a look is to determine for what occasion the make-up is to be created. Is she interested in a general corrective make-up, one for every day wear, or is it for that special evening out?

For daytime it is usually best to strive for a natural look. It depends of course on the type of client you are working on. Needless to say, a glamourous type will wear more make-up than the outdoor type. In either case, the make-up should still be done with the fact in mind that daylight will show up every facet of the make-up application and it should be applied subtlely.

For evening, colors may be intensified, application somewhat exaggerated and frosted or pearlized products will add their own luster and excitement.

FACIAL SHAPE

The fourth step for designing a look is a careful study of the facial shape. It is not necessary to attempt to make every shape appear to be the ideal oval. It is necessary, however, to give it its most attractive contour, hide any of its flaws and to sculpture the features to give them their most attractive appearance.

COMPLEXION QUALITY

The fifth step is to now take note of the complexion. If it is smoothly textured, it needs only a fine application of base to even out the skin tone. A flawed complexion, on the other hand, may require a heavier and more opaque make-up base application to smooth out its texture. Too heavy a make-up application, however, can do the opposite and actually accentuate lines and problem areas of the skin, so it is important to adjust the base to the individual.

Chapter 4

Preparation for the Make-up Application

It is not necessary to invest a great deal of money to set up a make-up area, but rather to design an area that wisely utilizes the space available for maximum effectiveness. Keeping the area spotlessly clean and as attractive as possible will give the desired professional look to the entire endeavor. If the make-up area is part of a beauty salon, a curtained booth or a room away from the main area of the salon should be available for individual make-up lessons. Simple make-up applications may be done in an open area to encourage other clients to take advantage of the make-up services.

The basic necessities for a make-up center are:

1. A cosmetic cabinet for both display and storage.

2. A make-up vanity with a large clear mirror.

3. A make-up chair with a headrest that can recline and adjust to height.

4. A good lighting system.

ADJUSTING THE CLIENT'S HAIR

The preparation you make for the make-up application depends on the individual situation. If the client has had her hair set in the salon, the correct time to do the make-up is after she comes out of the dryer, or after the hair has been blown-dry. Merely place out of the way any strands that may be set onto the face or forehead.

After completing the make-up service the stylist may then do the combout. As an added bonus you will find that the client will invariably admire her coiffure all the more when she sees it as a frame for the more attractive face reflected in the mirror.

If the client is not having her hair done, but merely her face made-up, it is only necessary to brush any hair away from the face. You may find it necessary to pin or clip the hair back so that it will not interfere with your work. The hair is only covered with a towel or hair band when doing a facial or on some special occasion, such as when photographing a step-by-step make-up procedure. It stands to reason that if a client comes to the salon for just a make-up service and has her hairstyle disturbed with a hair covering she will expect you to take the time to put it back into its former state. This will waste your time and not always work out successfully.

Use an attractive make-up cape to protect the client's dress. If the cape is used continuously on various people then it is wise to use a neck strip first for sanitary purposes.

POSITIONING THE CLIENT

Keep the client in an upright position when applying make-up. It is preferable to use a headrest for comfort, tilting the chair only slightly backwards. If the client is allowed to lie in a horizontal position while being made-up, the facial structure will be in a different alignment, making correction of facial problems such as under-eye shadows, mouth lines, and jowls, difficult to correct.

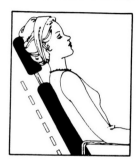

Position for make-up application

When the client is receiving make-up instructions, she should sit upright and be somewhat closer to the mirror. This would obviously preclude the use of the headrest.

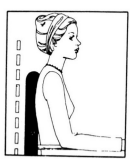

Position for make-up instructions

For applying creams and massaging, you may stand behind the client. At all other times you should stand on one side of the client without moving from one side to the other. The right-handed make-up artist should stand on the right side of the client, and the left-handed artist should stand and work from the left side.

When working without a headrest, do not allow the client to tilt her head too far back as to cause discomfort, but rather raise the chair to accommodate your height and convenience.

Remember not only to check your client as you work at close range, but also to check the make-up in the mirror for distance and perspective.

SKIN PREPARATION

It is important that the skin be prepared properly before application of any make-up. The skin must be cleansed thoroughly, toned, and protected with a moisturizer. These are the three basic steps that are suggested both prior to the make-up application and for removal of the make-up before bedtime or after a theatrical presentation.

Cleanser

Depending on the type of skin you are working on and the amount of make-up to be removed, you may choose to use a mild liquid cleansing milk or a heavier type of cleansing cream used for removing theatre make-up. Having pinned the forehead and side hair out of the way, dot the cleanser all over the face, including the forehead, cheeks, eyelids, nose and chin. With small circular movements of the fingertips, massage the cleanser into the skin to help lift off the old cosmetics and dirt.

Special areas may be cleansed as follows:

1. To cleanse the **upper-eye area,** have the client close her eyes and hold the lid taut by drawing the skin upward at the brow bone. Rub very gently back and forth with the fingertips of the other hand to loosen eye make-up and mascara. To remove extra-heavy eye make-up you may use eye make-up remover pads or lightly saturate a cotton pad with mineral oil and apply to the eye area. The only drawback to the mineral oil is that it must be removed thoroughly or it will break down the fresh eye make-up to be applied.

2. To cleanse the **under-eye area,** have the client open her eyes and look upward. Draw the skin taut at the outer corner of the eyes and rub gently back and forth with fingertips under the eye.

3. To remove **lipstick** apply some cleanser to a tissue and remove all excess lipcolor by stroking from the outer corner toward the center of the lips.

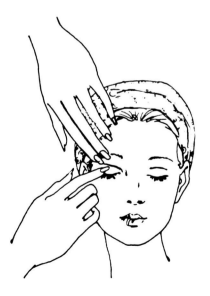

Hand position on upper-eye area

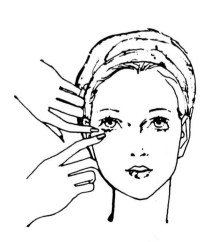

Hand position on under-eye area

To remove the cleanser, fold a tissue and begin at the center of the face. Wipe the tissue outward to the hairline, being careful not to get cleanser on the hair. Start on the forehead, then the nose and cheek area, and then the chin and neck. All manipulations on the face should be in an upward and outward direction; never drag the skin down. With a fresh tissue, clean the eyelids and the under-eye areas holding the skin taut in the same manner as when applying the cleanser. Cleanse the lips again in the same manner as before, using cleanser on a tissue. If there is still a certain amount of lip stain left that you wish to remove you may do so with the eye make-up remover pads or with the mineral oil.

Cotton pads, saturated with water and then rung out, may be used for removing the cleanser on very sensitive skins.

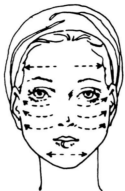

Cleansing movements

Toners

Toners are basically astringents in liquid form, that are used to help remove all traces of cleanser, close the pores and tone and stimulate the skin. You should have a mild, non-alcoholic skin freshener for normal to dry skins, and a stronger astringent for the normal to oily types. To apply toner, saturate a pledget of cotton with the toner. Pat it briskly on the skin for stimulation, then rub gently from the center of the face with long strokes outward to the hairline. Repeat this step with a clean pledget of cotton if necessary. All traces of cleanser must be removed. In general it is best to avoid the eye area when using astringents.

Moisturizer

One of the most important steps in preparing the skin for a flawless make-up application is to coat the skin with a fine film of moisturizer. This is done to help:

1. Keep the moisture balance of the skin at its proper level

2. Fight dry lines, and the flaking present on dry skin

3. Assist in even application of make-up.

To apply the moisturizer, dot the moisturizer onto the areas that need attention the most: the outer area of the eyes, the mouth area, the forehead and the neck. Massage into the skin with small firm circular movements. If desired, you may stand behind the client and using the fingertips of both hands, massage the moisturizer into the skin with upward and outward strokes.

All traces of the moisturizer must be absorbed by the skin. That which is not, should be blotted with a tissue. To check for any residual traces of moisturizer left on the surface, stroke the sides of the face with the back of your hands; if it feels satiny smooth, then the skin is ready for the application of make-up. Actually it is preferable to use less rather than too much moisturizer under make-up.

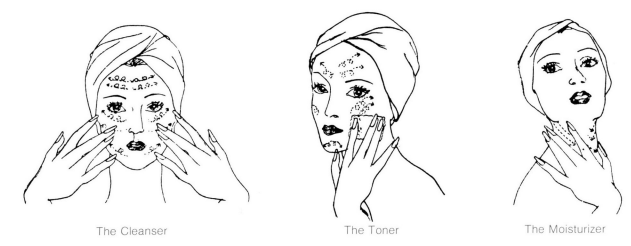

The Cleanser   The Toner   The Moisturizer

Application and removal of skin care products is always done with an upward and outward direction except on the neck area. For this area, the head is tilted back to tauten the neck and the movement is downward.

DESIGNING THE EYEBROW

The brow design must be decided upon at the time of your initial evaluation of your customer's individual make-up needs and before any make-up is applied to the face. If the brow line is not good, it can often be reshaped somewhat by plucking. If this is insufficient, further reshaping can be done with the brow pencil. If the brow is well-formed and well-placed, it need only be darkened or more clearly defined. The object in this case is to darken only the brow hairs, not the skin.

Classic brow design

The classic brow design is as follows:

1. The brow should start above the inner corner of the eye.

2. The high point of the arch should be somewhere between the outer edge of the iris and the outer corner of the eye.

3. You will find where to end the brow by slanting a pencil from the side of the nose to the outer corner of the eye to the brow line.

4. The beginning and end of the eyebrow should be at approximately the same level.

Classic
brow design

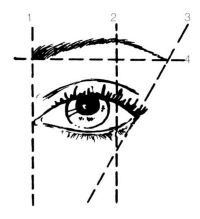

23

Shaping the brow

Any plucking that needs to be done should be done after the skin has been cleansed and before the toner is applied. Usually only the hairs on the under side of the brow are removed, since you will, in most cases, wish to increase the space between the lash line and the brow line. If, however, you wish to lower the brows or lessen the angle of the arch, you may carefully remove some of the upper hairs. In all cases, you must avoid giving the brows a too clearly defined look, since this will give a hard look to the eyes and appear artificial. In filling out brows which are sparse, or to extend them, use a soft crayon pencil which is the same color as the brows and has an extremely fine point. Lightly sketch in lines which will approximate the hairs of the brow itself. Remember, plucking is done before make-up and penciling is done afterwards.

A well-proportioned eyebrow is thickest at the inner portions, slenderizes toward the arch, and tapers off at the end. Each face calls for an individual approach to brow design. Basically, the eyebrow should be proportioned to the basic facial structure with a heavy-featured face having a stronger, more pronounced brow than a delicately featured face.

Brow shapes for certain face shapes and any ideas you may have of the "classic" brow shape should be modified to reflect current fashion trends. It should be remembered, though, that even when you are adhering to the most current brow fashion, you must make some changes in your design to suit a customer with a particular problem.

Procedure for shaping

1. Place the customer back in a reclining position with head supported by a head rest.

2. Cleanse the brows with cleansing cream.

3. Wipe off all traces of cream.

4. Stretch the area to be tweezed between the thumb and forefinger.

5. Pluck the hairs in the same direction as the hair growth.

6. Clean all straggling hair from the underside of the brow.

7. Make sure the brow bone is clean of hairs; this is important so that when eye-shadows are applied they will go on smoothly.

8. The top area of the eyebrow is tweezed when major changes are to be made.

9. When tweezing is finished, apply skin freshener or astringent to the area.

Chapter 5

Corrective Make-up Techniques

Bone structure determines facial shape while cartilage and muscle determine the planes, contours and features of the face. It is, therefore, possible only by drastic means, such as plastic surgery, to change the basic structure of someone's face. There are, however, many steps that may be taken to create the illusion of a more appealing facial shape and contour than that with which one was born. These illusions are created by various methods such as the length, shape and style of one's hair but even more effectively by make-up application.

With the aid of cosmetics, it is possible to create various effects and illusions which result in a more harmonious symmetry to facial features and a more attractive contour to the face. Facial sculpturing and contouring is achieved by the **Chiaroscuro technique** which has long been used as a classic technique in theatrical make-up and has become popular in corrective, fashion and in evening make-up.

CHIAROSCURO MAKE-UP TECHNIQUES

Chiaroscuro is a word that should be prominent in the vocabulary of anyone remotely involved with make-up whether as a make-up artist, teacher or salesperson.

The word chiaroscuro means, literally, light and shade. The principles of chiaroscuro have been used by painters for centuries and today the same principles are applied to photography and make-up application. Basically, the chiaroscuro technique rests on principles of light and shadow and that the way light falls on an object determines how it is seen. The amount of light and the direction from which it comes, as well as the color of the light determines how any object appears to the eye. An example of this is the sparkle of a diamond; it may only glitter in the dimness of moonlight, but brilliantly sparkle when seen in the full light of the sun. When light falls on a three dimensional object the most prominent areas reflect the most light and thus appear larger, while the adjacent areas that are more in shadow appear smaller. Knowledge of these principles and the techniques to follow are indispensable to the successful make-up artist.

Contouring and sculpturing

Through the use of highlighting and shading cosmetics, the make-up artist literally attempts to emphasize or alter the contours of the facial features and indeed the general outline of the face. In this manner one might say we are sculpturing the features and contouring the face. The proper application of cosmetics can actually add a lovely sculptured appearance to the eyes, nose and cheek bones. The words contouring and sculpturing therefore are somewhat interchangeable.

Contour creams when utilized for sculpturing a feature or contouring the face, are used directly after the application of make-up base and before powdering the face.

Highlighting and shading powders are often in pressed cake form and should be applied with a brush after the make-up base has been set with a basic translucent powder. Highlighters are often pearlized.

All contouring must be done very carefully, and all shaded or highlighted areas blended so that no line of demarcation is visible. Shading for daytime make-up must be applied with extreme care. Highlighting on the other hand, may be used more freely. If you wish, you may use only highlighting and let the other areas automatically fall into shadow and appear to recede.

It is the unusual face which requires extensive corrective make-up or recontouring. This is usually done in theatrical make-up when the change must be a dramatic one. It is more often the case that only one area or feature needs sculpting or correcting. Here are some suggestions for the reshaping of various facial features although, in practice, you will probably devise methods of your own. Every face is different and one method will not suit all.

Highlighting and shading

The basic principle of this technique is the use of light and shadow to create a dimensional effect. Any object that is highlighted will reflect light, come into greater prominence, and appear larger. Conversely, an object that is darker than its background will seem smaller and appear to recede. Thus, a light tone used on the cheek bone and a darker shade below it will give that area a hollow look. In this manner a dimensional effect will be achieved. When this technique is used by applying only shading and highlighting and a minimum of color, a striking and dramatic look can be achieved.

Highlighting may be accomplished with any light-tinted product in a cream or powdered form and preferably in an ivory, beige, or off-white shade.

Shading cream or powder may be brown, gray-brown, or mauve colors with natural shadowing qualities.

Other products used for sculpting and contouring are:

1. Pearlized creams and liquids for highlighting.

2. Deep-toned blushers for shading.

3. Loose pearlized powders for glowing effects.

Similar effects can also be achieved with color, using the same technique, but only if the colors are lighter or darker than the overall tone of the skin. For example, a bright pink blusher used on the fullness of the cheek bone will bring that area into prominence and a deep mauve blusher used below the cheek bone will deepen that area and give it a more hollowed look.

Contouring the eyes with color follows a similar procedure. An area which you may wish to accentuate such as the eyelid or the brow bone may be tinted, let us say, with a pastel blue eye-shadow, while the center area above the crease line might be deepened with a darker blue or perhaps a dark plum-colored shadow.

Shiny and matte finishes

It is also possible to contour with alternating shiny and matte (dull) finished surfaces. A too large appearing nose may be diminished somewhat by powdering it into a matte finish, whereas a brow bone or cheek bone may be brought into greater prominence with the use of a pearlescent or glowing finish make-up base or powder.

Obviously, a light area with a shine will be more prominent than a light finish which is matte. A shadowed matte finish, by the same principle, will appear deeper than a dark shade that has a glow to it, since a shiny surface will reflect light and a dull surface will tend to absorb it. You can also contour a face by using two make-up bases of the same color and finish but with different degrees of depth or value. Examples would be the use of pale beige and a dark beige, or creamy pink and a dusty rose tone. In actual practice, when slenderizing a round face, the lighter color would be used in the center of the face and the darker tones on the side, blending them together where they meet.

CONCEALING FLAWS

To achieve the perfect make-up and a look of a flawless complexion, more often than not you will find it necessary to do a certain amount of corrective work. This type of make-up is used to diminish or conceal complexion flaws. Common complexion flaws include under-eye shadows, eye circles, blemishes, moles, birthmarks and wrinkles.

To conceal flaws, it is necessary to use an opaque cream somewhat heavier than the foundation or base. If the cover-up is to be applied under the base, the cream may be a light beige shade. This shade may be used on any tone of skin from the lightest to the darkest, since the foundation will tint the entire face to an even color. When used over the base, the cover-up should be closer to the skin color. In any case, the cream must always be somewhat lighter than the make-up base.

The most effective method of applying the cover-up is with a corrective brush. For ease of application, brush the cover-up on in small areas and carefully blend with the fingertips leaving on just enough to cover flaws and unwanted shadows. Any excess cover-up which is left on the skin will create the impression of a flaw. In any event, it is important to avoid an excessive build-up of make-up. When applying the make-up base over the corrected areas, pat it on gently so that the cover-up is not wiped away. A corrective cream is ideal for concealing under-eye shadows, eye circles, blemishes, moles, birthmarks and wrinkles.

The under-eye area

Practically everyone has some problem or flaw in the under-eye area which needs correction or concealment. The most common flaws in this area are dark shadows or puffiness. Contrary to popular belief, these conditions are due neither to dissipation nor lack of sleep. Under-eye problems are usually a natural part of the aging process or an inherited trait. Though not usually caused by systemic problems or dissipation, they will be aggravated by certain illnesses and by fatigue. Lack of sufficient rest will certainly add to the problem but, oddly enough, too much sleep will often have a tendency to accentuate puffiness under and over the eyes; this is due to fluids accumulating in the tissues while the body is in a horizontal position. During the course of the day, the fluids will drain away and the puffiness will diminish.

To correct the under-eye puff, the dark shadow or circle below the protuberance of this puff should be lightened and not the puff itself. Another technique used on puffs which require more skillful application is to use a slightly deeper shade of foundation on the puff and the lighter cover-up in the shadow. Then blend the two together carefully, thus equalizing the puffed and shadow areas.

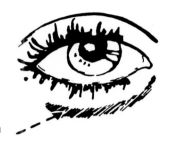

Concealing
under-eye area

Circles

A more common problem is a dark shadowed area below the eyes. To eradicate this shadow, you may apply the cover-up to the entire area in a thin application always feathering the edges.

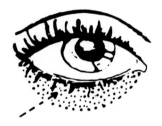

Concealing
circles

Blemishes and moles

Blemishes and moles should be touched-up carefully, applying the cream with a brush. It may have to be retouched after the foundation has been applied.

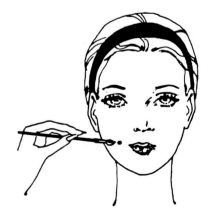

Concealing
blemishes

Birthmarks

When covering a birthmark that encompasses a larger area, the cover-up may be applied first, powdered lightly with a translucent powder, and touched-up with another application of cover-up, if necessary. The make-up base is then feathered on delicately to avoid moving the underlying corrective work.

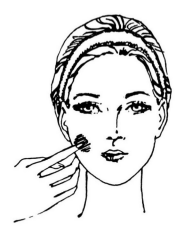

Concealing
birthmarks

Wrinkles

Frown lines, wrinkles, and the naso-labial fold (nose-to-mouth lines) may be diminished by using a cover-up cream. A highlighting cream, however, may prove more effective since it has more reflective properties. Every line or fold has a shadow in the depth of the crease. Using a brush, apply the highlighter in a very thin line directly into the line or wrinkle. Smooth off the excess with the fingertips and then, stretching out the skin, dust over with translucent powder. Remove all excess powder to avoid a build-up of make-up which will accentuate the lines rather than diminish them.

The ultimate aim is to achieve as smooth and flawless a complexion as possible. There are, however, limitations to what can be accomplished with cosmetics.

Remember that it is possible to use too much make-up or to use it incorrectly which will result in undesired effects. A thin application of corrective products and the lightest possible touch of powder will offer the most rewarding results.

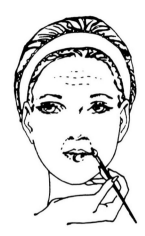

Concealing
wrinkles

DESIGNING THE EYE

In making-up the eyes you must be concerned with giving them the most attractive shape possible. This is done using the cosmetics in a manner that is the most contemporary and, when necessary, contouring and reshaping them to bring them into harmony with the total look of beauty you wish to achieve.

Simple corrective work with cosmetics, using color, highlighting, shading, and liner will go far to minimize defects and create a more pleasing effect. The proper sequence of application of eye make-up is as follows:

1. Eye-shadows

2. Eye-liner

3. Curl lashes (if eyelash curler is used)

4. Mascara

5. Eyebrow pencil

EYE-SHADOW AND EYE-LINER

Eye-shadows

Without eye-shadow even the most beautiful or striking eyes can lose much of their brilliance and effectiveness. With the improper application of eye-shadow, the importance of the eyes as the focal point of interest on the face can be greatly diminished. It is, therefore, of the utmost importance that you, as a professional make-up artist, perfect your artistry in the use of eye-shadows. You must learn all the various uses of these products, the different effects that can be created, and all the subtle nuances which you can utilize to achieve just the "look" that you may be striving for.

Eye-shadows come in a great variety of colors and finishes. Here are some of the different types of eye-shadow products available:

Pressed-powder shadow: Applied with a sponge applicator or brush, this type of eye-shadow is simple to apply and will not separate on the lid.

Wet and dry shadow: This pressed-powder shadow goes on dry for a soft tint effect or is brushed in with water for a more intensified color.

Cream shadow: Although the simplest of all to apply, this shadow may separate in the lid creases.

Emulsion cream shadow: This water-based cream shadow strokes on smoothly as a cream but dries somewhat; it will not separate on the lid as much as the regular cream or stick shadows do.

There are, of course, many other types of products each of which has individual characteristics. The above are among the more popular types of eye-shadows used.

The following hints should be kept in mind when applying eye-shadows:

- If you are using cream eye-shadows, they should be applied before powdering the face.

- Most people find the powdered eye-shadows much easier to use. This type of eye-shadow is to be applied after the face is powdered.

- Use matte eye-shadows for most color, contouring and shading.

- Pearlized shadows are best used for dramatic purposes and evening wear. Remember that pearlized products have a tendencey to accentuate flaws and will emphasize puffiness, lines and crepey eyelids.

- For shading and contouring use colors such as brown, charcoal, umber, mocha, navy, and other colors with shading qualities.

- For highlighting use ivory, pink, beige, peach and other soft, light colors.

Eye-liners

As the master key to shaping or reshaping the eye, no one product is as diversified as eye-liner. It can accentuate the eye, change its shape and size, and make the eyelashes appear thicker and more lush. A skillful application of eye-liner can even help create the illusion of more evenly spaced and set eyes and thus give a better balance to the entire face.

Some types of eye-liner products are:

Lining pencils or crayons: Pencils are excellent for outlining the eyes for both regular use and for photography. These are easy to apply, can be soft or strong looking depending on the application and are easy to blend. They are also the only safe type of cosmetic for use on the inside of the lid assuming they are approved for this purpose.

Cake eye-liner: This type of liner is most used by the professional for stage work because of its diversity and long lasting qualities. It is applied with a dampened fine line brush and the depth and intensity of color can be varied by the amount of water used.

Liquid eye-liner: The merits of liquid eye-liner are that it is long lasting and that it usually comes in a bottle with its own brush. Under ordinary circumstances though, one cannot obtain any variation in the depth of the shade and the brush cannot give as fine a line as one can obtain with cake liner.

Colors used may be dark brown, black, charcoal and navy.

Contouring the eye: eye-shadow and eye-liner application

Eyelids should be dry before eye-shadows are applied. If powdered eye-shadow is to be used, it is wise to first powder the lids lightly with translucent powder.

Have the client look down with her eyes almost closed, then, with the fingers of one hand on the brow bone, draw the lid lightly upward to hold the skin taut. Now apply the shadow from the inner corner of the lid to the outer corner with the strongest application of color at the base of the lashes. Always blend your colors upward and outward.

When contouring the eye, use the technique of highlighting and shading to achieve the best results. As a general rule follow this manner of application:

1. As a base use a light shade of matte eye-shadow over the entire eyelid area.

2. Use your shading color for contouring the depth area which is the center area directly above the eyelid crease.

3. If you are going to use an accent eye color on the lid, apply it now.

4. A highlighting shadow can be used now where desired.

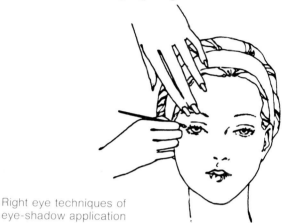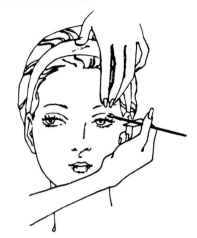

Right eye techniques of eye-shadow application

Left eye

Described below are some popular eye designs:

1. CONSERVATIVE: This is the most popularly used eye design. A shading color contours the depth area and blends outward and somewhat upward giving the eye a slight lift. A color accent may be used on the lid itself and wraps around the lower corner of the eye to form a color frame for the eyes. A fine eye-line is drawn on the upper lid at the base of the lashes to delineate the eye shape. Lower liner starts one third out from the inner corner extending to the outer corner.

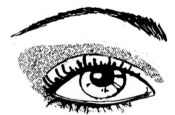

Conservative

2. CLASSIC: This fashionable and popular eye contour is also an effective design for a slightly drooping lid. Shading shadow starts at the center of the eye contouring the depth area and blends outward. It then comes around the outer corner of the eye to form a horizontal V-shape. Eye-liner starts on the upper lid near the inner corner in a very fine line until it passes the center portion of the eye. It is then made to thicken to a pointed wedge shape as it reaches the outer corner. Lower liner is thinner and meets the upper liner at the outer corner.

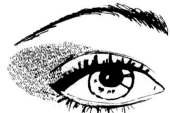

Classic

3. ROUND: For a wide-eyed innocent look the round eye is most appropriate. A rounded contouring shadow accentuates the center or depth area. Accent color may be applied to the eyelid itself, and a highlighter may be used on the brow bone if desired. Liner on the upper lid starts very thin at the inner corner and widens at the center of the eye then tapers again to a very thin line ending at the outer corner. Bottom liner may be used in a similar manner but much finer and softer.

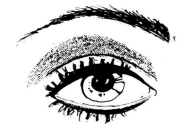

Round

4. OBLIQUE: This eye shape is a favorite of those who prefer an exotic look. All movement has an oblique or slanted direction giving an almond shape to the eye. A medium shade of shadow is brushed upward at the inner part of the eyelid. A deeper value of the same color moves outward drawing the eye upward at the outer area. Liner on the upper lid starts quite thin at the inner corner and draws steadily wider as it approaches the outer corner where it extends outward in an oblique line. Lower liner is drawn up to meet the upper eye at the outer corner.

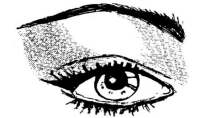

Oblique

5. OPEN END: This eye design is ideal for the small eye in that it delineates the eye without closing it in. An accent color may be applied to the eyelid area up to the crease line. A deeper shading color sweeps from there to the brow leaving a highlight on the brow bone. Eye-liner is applied in a sweeping stroke from the inner corner out past the outer portion of the eye. Lower liner is a thinner version of the upper liner, both curving out past the outside without meeting.

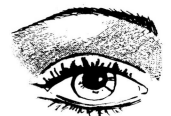

Open End

MASCARA

If a woman wears no make-up other than lipstick and mascara, she can, at a glance, appear to be fully made-up. The reason for this is that she has emphasized the two major focal points of her face.

The use of mascara as a frame for the eyes will increase their dramatic qualities, define their shape and size, and intensify their depth and color. Mascara will also make the lashes appear longer and thicker particularly if, as is usually the case, the lashes are lighter at the tips than they are at the base. The lashes should curl up so their fringe-like qualities will be most effective.

Types of mascara

The two most popular types of mascara are:

Cake mascara: This mascara is applied with a small brush and water and, because it is mixed, can be used in varying degrees of consistency.

Applicator mascara wand: This type of mascara is preferred by most women for personal use since it is self-contained and is easily carried in the purse.

When choosing a mascara color, keep in mind that black mascara may be used on most women to good effect. Brown mascara is effective for those with very pale hair and lashes. Shades such as blue or green may be used for special effect or to coordinate with eye-shadow colors.

Mascara application

Mascara is applied after eye-shadow and eye-liner, but before false lashes if they are going to be used.

Apply mascara to the lower lashes first and then the upper lashes. For the lower lashes, have the client look upward and stroke on the mascara carefully, making sure not to get it on the skin. If it does smear onto the skin, wipe it off quickly with a dry Q-tip. When using the mascara wand, always hold it horizontally in line with the eyes.

When applying mascara to the upper lashes, have the client look down, eyes open about half way. If necessary, you may place your thumb on the brow bone and gently stretch the skin upward. This will make the lashes more accessible and also help to keep them separated. Begin applying mascara at the outer corner of the eye as close to the base of the lashes as possible without touching the skin and draw the brush gently upward on the lashes from the base to the tips. Using the same method, work your way inward until all the lashes have been coated with a fine layer of mascara.

Repeat this procedure several times, allowing each application to dry before the next layer is applied. In this way, you will gradually build up color and thickness on the lashes while maintaining a smooth, even finish. Care should be exercised when applying mascara to prevent the lashes from sticking to each other and having a matted look. An eyelash brush or comb may be used between each mascara application to help keep the lashes separated.

ARTIFICIAL EYELASHES

Although artificial lashes are a sometimes thing in fashion, they are a useful adjunct to make-up in various situations. Actresses on stage often use them, as do showgirls who consider them a must. Short, somewhat curly lashes are useful for make-up on the mature eye where an overhanging eyelid precludes the use of much eye-shadow or liner. Natural looking lashes give this type of eye a much needed lift. Oriental women often have very short lashes and too can benefit from the use of false lashes.

The look you wish to achieve will determine the type of lashes you select for each individual make-up. They must, of course, complement the make-up rather than distract from or in any way diminish the overall look you are striving for.

Fitting the lashes

To look and feel natural, eyelashes must be fitted correctly. After removing the lashes from the platform, (carefully, so as not to pull them apart), place the lash against the base of the real lashes, positioning it about a third of an inch away from the inner corner of the eye. Since strip lashes are usually a bit wider than the eyelid, you will find that the lash extends past the outer corner of the eye. It is this extra bit of lash that will have to be cut off.

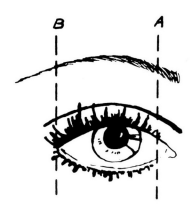

Fitting the lash

Trimming the lashes

Remove the lash from the eye and trim off the excess from the outer end. This will leave the inner corner of the lashes short and the outer end longer. Should you wish to have a rounded eye look, you may trim off the excess from the inner corner.

If the lash hairs are too long, they may be shortened with a pair of manicuring scissors. Do not cut them off straight across, but rather cut into the tips of the lashes to give an uneven, natural tapered line. In other words, some hairs will be shorter than others, as your own lashes are.

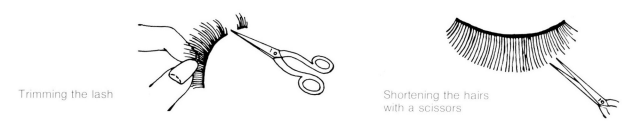

Trimming the lash

Shortening the hairs with a scissors

Feathering the lashes

If you want to be very professional, a really good job can be done by feathering the lashes with a single-edged razor blade. Place the lash face down on a smooth, hard surface (the box the lashes come in is a good choice) and flatten it out by holding it down with the forefinger of one hand. Holding the razor in the other hand, straight up and down rather than angled, feather the lashes with a scraping, outward stroke, again making some lashes shorter than others.

Cutting or feathering the lashes should be done only when necessary. If possible, it is preferable to choose a lash with hairs that are just the desired length and fullness for the individual client's needs.

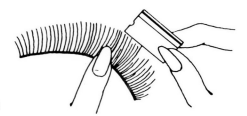
Feathering the lashes

Curling lashes

To curl the lash, dampen it and lay it on a piece of tissue. Wrap the tissue around a pencil and let it dry. Another method is to use an eyelash curler on the dry lash.

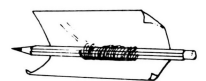
Curling the lash

Lashes in groups

If you choose just to use a few groups of lashes or if you wish to attain a spikey or feathery-eyed look, cut lashes into small groups of from two to six hairs. These are applied at intervals to the base of the lashes with adhesive. These can be used both on the top and bottom lashes applying the longer hairs in larger groups to the top, and the smaller and finer groups as bottom lashes.

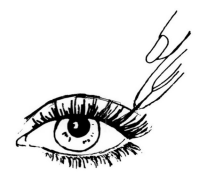
Lashes in groups

Applying the adhesive

Use a good surgical lash adhesive and apply it directly from the tube, being careful to use only a very small amount. Hold the lash in one hand with a pair of tweezers while applying the adhesive. Avoid getting the adhesive on the hairs and apply it only to the base or band of the eyelash. It is actually best to use a toothpick to apply the adhesive. This will avoid the possibility of too heavy an application.

Eyelashes will be easier to apply if they are shaped to fit the curve of the eye. As soon as adhesive is on, hold the lash in a horseshoe form for a few seconds. This will give the adhesive a little time to become tacky and at the same time give form to the lash.

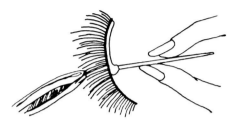

Applying adhesive with a toothpick

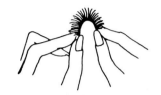

Shaping the lash

Applying the lashes

Have the client look down or close her eyes. If her eyelid has a tendency to flutter, draw the skin of the eyelid taut by lifting the skin at the brow bone. Holding the lash with a tweezer, place it against the eye as close to the base of the natural lash as possible. Remember to keep it at least a third of an inch away from the inner corner and end it at the outer corner of the eye. When it is in place, press down all along the band with the back end of the tweezer to adhere it firmly to the lid.

Now press the real lashes and the false lashes together, with either the tweezer or with your thumb and forefinger, to help them blend.

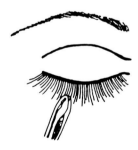

Applying the lash with a tweezer

Corrective lash application

For corrective lash application, take note of the following tips:

- **Deep-set eyes:** Use long, very fine lashes on an invisible base. These will have a tendency to bring the eyes forward and out from under the brow bone.

- **Close-set eyes:** Cut lashes to half or demi size and place them just before the center of the eye and out slightly past the outer corner of the eyes.

- **Down-turned eyes:** Eyes that slant downward at the outer corners can be lifted by placing the outer edge of the lash slightly above the natural lash base.

- **Protruding eyes:** Heavy lashes would only emphasize the lid fullness. It is best to use very natural, fairly short lashes. The lash should be longest at the outer corner to give the eye a lengthened rather than a rounded look.

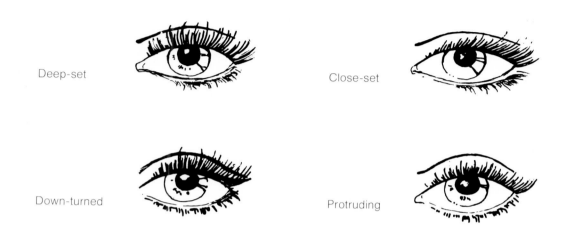

Deep-set   Close-set

Down-turned   Protruding

Removal and care of lashes

1. Lashes should be removed by grasping the outer part of the lash and peeling it off toward the inner corner.

2. The adhesive is removed by holding the lash in one hand and peeling the adhesive off gently in one strip. Be very careful not to harm the lash itself.

3. If the mascara or adhesive is on the lash hairs then the lash must be cleaned. Use a lash cleaner or wig cleaner for this purpose. Drop the lash into the cleaner and leave it for a few minutes. Then remove it and place it on a towel.

EYEBROWS

The proper shape and correct position of the eyebrows are of the utmost importance in maintaining the overall balance of the face. Because of their mobility, the eyebrows can emphasize facial expressions and convey a vast range of moods and emotions. They can, thus, either increase or decrease the dramatic qualities of the eyes. The color and fullness of the brows are of equal importance. Heavy, well-defined brows, for example, would be best suited for a woman with large features, whereas they would be out of place on a small delicately chiseled face and create unwanted emphasis in that area.

Eyebrow products

Some types of eyebrow products are:

> **Brow pencil:** The best type of brow pencil should have a very thin lead point. To keep a fine point on pencils, you may use a pencil sharpener or a single-edged razor blade.

Brow pencils are best for filling in, shaping and extending the brows, and some may also be used for lining the eyes.

Brush-on brow coloring: This type of brow coloring comes in pressed-powder, compact form and has a firm, contoured brow brush for easy application. It is best when a soft, feathery, natural look is desired.

Brows suited to the individual

The shape of the brows depend upon the size, shape, and general contour of the woman's face, as well as upon the look that you wish to achieve. There is no one shape which is perfect for every woman. It is up to you to decide whether the natural shape of your customer's brows is the best shape for her individual look, or if you must alter it to her facial contours. In many cases you will find that, although a woman's brows are not what you would consider a perfect shape, they are right for her and add just the look of individuality. In these cases, you will need to concern yourself only with the position.

Brow color

Brow pencils should be used only when necessary, such as redesigning an arch, filling in empty spots or accentuating the shape or color of a brow. Choose a color close to the natural hair shade. For black hair go one shade lighter and for very light hair go one shade darker.

When sketching in the eyebrows where they are not full enough, merely fill in any little empty places with a pencil. When trying to compensate for really thin brows, sketch on the shape of the brow with a light brown pencil and then with a very sharp-pointed dark brown pencil sketch in tiny hairlike strokes within this shaping. For those who cannot master the brow pencil successfully a 'brush on brow' product may be easier to use.

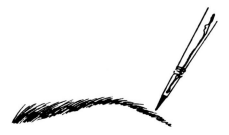

Adding brow color

SPECIAL EYE SHAPE CORRECTIONS

The following four eye types sometimes call for a special eye make-up application.

Prominent eyes

1. Prominent eyes will appear less protruding when shaded with a brown, gray, or deep plum tone of eye-shadow. The deepest color tone should be close to the lash line and fade gradually up to the brow bone. A matte-finish shadow is preferable; avoid those shadows which have a high sheen or pearlized finish.

39

2. If the brow bone is not too prominent, a highlighter may be used.

3. A thin line of eye-liner can be applied down at the lash base and extended outward slightly to detract somewhat from the roundness of the eye. Lower liner may be applied above the base of the lashes.

4. The brow should be slightly arched, not rounded and not exaggerated.

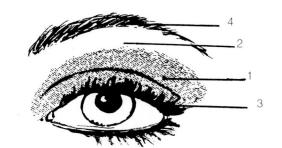

The prominent eye

Deep-set eyes

1. Increase the eyelid area by tweezing the brows from the underside and arch as high as possible.

2. Highlight the entire eyelid area with a highlighter or bright eye-shadow.

3. If the brow bone is too prominent, it may be shaded slightly to make it appear to recede.

4. Use a thin lower liner applied slightly below the base of the lashes and extended outward past the outer eye corner. Fill in this corner area with a highlighter to give an open-eye effect.

5. The use of very thin, long lashes can do much to bring the eyes out. The base of these lashes should be very fine. The liner on the upper lid is very thin.

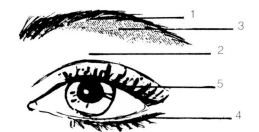

Deep-set eyes

Drooping eyes

To offset the droop of the eye which is often accompanied by a low bone structure or a low lid fold, it is necessary to give the appearance of a lift to the entire eye area.

1. Tweeze the under area of the outer portion of the brow to allow a better arch.

2. Shading shadow is applied across the fold and smudged outward and upward.

3. Highlighter is placed directly under the arch of the brow.

4. Eye-liner is applied in a very thin line and thickened slightly at the outside in a wedgelike point to give a lift to the eye.

5. Lower liner, when used, is applied in a straight line and then brought up at the outer corner.

6. If lashes are used, they should be applied slightly higher at the outer corner of the eyes.

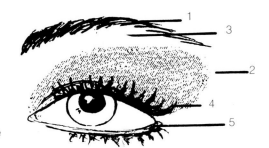

Correcting the drooping eye

Close-set eyes

1. Tweeze brows slightly past the inner corner of eyes and bring them out well past the eyes' outer corners.

2. Apply a highlighter or lightly toned eye-shadow such as beige at the inner area of the eye.

3. Colored eye-shadow should start near the center of the eye and should extend outward past the outer eye area.

4. Both upper and lower eye-liners should start past the inner corner and extend outward from the outer corner of the eye.

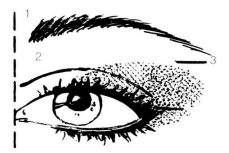

Correcting
close-set eyes

BLUSHING THE SKIN

Adding color highlights to the skin gives life and interest to the face. Without these tints, the face should be the flat, unrelieved tone of the foundation. It is blush (rouge) that gives vibrancy to the skin and added luster to the eyes.

Types of blushes

There are various types of blushes. Some of the most popular forms are:

Cream blush: Applied directly over the foundation, it adds creamy color, with some sheen, and has long lasting properties.

Pressed-powder blush: Applied after powder, it adds color and has a matte finish. It is ideal for touch-ups during the day. Some are pearlized and will add shine also.

The color is usually applied to the fullness of the cheek area. However, it can also be used in sculpting the face and to give a general color glow to the skin.

Blush, as an accent, may be used for highlighting and shading, depending on the shade and depth of its color.

Highlighting: Bright shades may be used as highlighters. For light skin the best shades are pink, peach, coral, orange, and red. For dark skin use tawny, bronze, coral, and red. When blush is used as a highlighter it attracts attention to that particular area and brings it into focus.

Shading: Deeper and more earthy tones have shading qualities. For light skin, shading blushes are tawny, mauve, and plum. For dark skin, deep bronze, dark plum, and wine are good. When blush is used for its shading qualities, the areas where it is applied will fall into shadow and appear to recede. When the skin has been shaded with a brown or gray-brown cream shader, it is often advisable to brush over these areas with a powdered blush to give the area a little color tone. This is done after the skin has been powdered with a translucent powder.

Application of cheek blush

To simplify the placement of the blush when used in cream form, it is best to apply it with the tips of the fingers in three dots within the area where it is to be blended. First, dot on the cream in a triangular pattern and then blend lightly and quickly with deft strokes upward and outward, skillfully blending the edges to leave no line of demarcation.

For Normal Placement—Blush goes directly on the cheek bone area and blends up toward the temples.

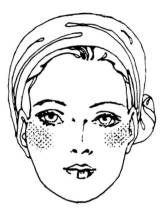

Normal
placement

For Round or Square Facial Shapes—If the face is round, wide or square, bring the rouge closer toward the nose, in an area directly under the center of the eye and blend up and out.

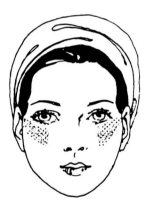

Round or
square face

For Oblong Facial Shapes—For an oblong-shaped face start the rouge slightly lower on the cheek area and blend from a line under the outer corner of the eye out toward the side of the face.

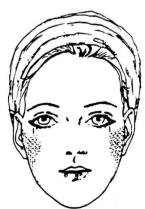

Oblong
face

Highlighting with blush

In order to give color dimension to the skin, particularly with beige or sallow skins, a technique called "blushing the skin" is used. The highlighting colors are used most often for this, although the tawny or bronze colors may be used on certain dark beige or tan skin tones for this purpose. Four areas for applying the blusher are: 1) on cheek bones 2) across forehead to temples, 3) on the brow bone, and 4) on the chin.

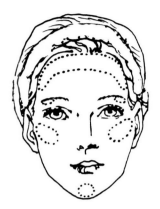

Highlighting
with blush

Shadowing with blush

The tawny or brownish-mauve shade of blush is used chiefly for shading the face. A pressed-powder type of shading rouge is particularly good for this purpose. It is best used under the cheek bones (in the hollows of the cheek) to accentuate the cheek bones and to create a more slenderized facial contour. The nose too can be slenderized with the use of this product, and the chin foreshortened. To apply, draw in the cheeks and brush shadow on under the cheek bones, from a point below the outer corner of the eye and up toward the ear. The strongest color delineation is in this area, then blend lightly onto cheek area and down slightly toward the jaw.

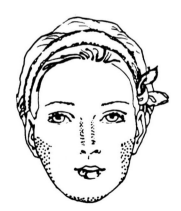

Shadowing
with blush

LIPS

The first step in the application of lip make-up is to outline the lips. This will give definition to their shape and serve as a guide for you in applying the color. The best results can be achieved with the use of a lip brush and a pencil. The brush is used after the liner to fill in the color on the lips. A lip pencil gives a fine, clear line which is less likely to smear. If the lips are outlined with a brush, the lips will have a less well-defined shape which, in some cases, may be desired. When outlining the lips with a pencil, use the same general shade as the lipstick you are going to apply to the mouth, but just a bit deeper in tone.

Application of lip color

1. The client's lips should be closed in a natural position, so that you can see the form being drawn on. Lean your small finger on the chin to steady your hand and start outlining the lips with the pencil. Do the upper lip first, starting from the lip corner away from you. Draw the line over the bow and then to the other corner. Now do the same for the lower lip.

2. Have the client open her lips and fill in the outer corner area.

3. With the lips drawn into a semi-smile and slightly parted, fill in with the lipstick, blending it again over the lip line that has been drawn in. This is particularly important where the color of the outline is darker than the rest of the lipstick. There should never be an obvious look of two separate shades, but rather a subtle blending.

Corrective lip make-up

A perfect lip line is an absolute necessity if the make-up is to be the most effective. You will find in many cases that the lip line needs correcting to some degree; examples are lips too full or too thin, an irregular lip line, a too thin upper lip or lower lip, or an entire lip line which is hazy and indistinct. In each case you must learn the correct technique to minimize these faults.

If you have properly evaluated your customer's make-up needs you will already have decided whether corrective work is to be done. Usually, the upper and lower lips should be of equal dimension. Since it is always easier to make a lip look thicker than thinner, it is better to fill out a thin lip, if necessary, rather than to attempt to make a full lip look thinner. Whatever is done must be with discretion, since alterations may be obvious, particularly where the natural lip line is very apparent.

Too thin lips: Use two shades of lip color. Outline slightly beyond the natural lip line with the deeper of the two shades. Fill in with the lighter shade and blend over the outline. Apply a lip gloss over all.

Outlining thin lips to make them fuller

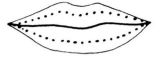

Too full lips: Apply a make-up base of cover-up to the mouth to camouflage the natural lip line. Use a lip color that is neither too bright nor too light in shade. A muted or earth tone lip color such as sienna or bronze is ideal. Draw the outline just inside the natural lip line and then fill in the lips. Avoid pearlescence or too much gloss.

Outlining full lips to make them thinner

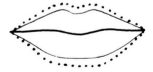

Too wide mouth: Avoid bringing the lip color to the corners of the mouth. If the lip is also thin, then give it a more rounded look by raising the bow of the upper lip and rounding out the lower lip. Use a gloss as a highlighter in the center of the lips only.

Outlining too-wide lips to make shorter

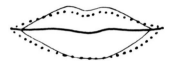

For corrective work, the use of two shades of lipstick can be extremely effective. If, for instance, the lips are disproportionate, a two-tone lipstick treatment will help to equalize them. When one lip is fuller than the other, use a bright color on the thinner lip and a duller shade on the fuller one. This will give an illusion of balance to the mouth.

When using two shades of lipstick, make sure that they are of related color value such as pink and red, coral and bronze, orange and brown, or merely a light and dark version of the same shade.

When less emphasis is desired on the mouth, lipstick may be blotted with a tissue to remove some of its luster and further de-emphasize the mouth.

Chapter 6

Face-Lifting Techniques for the Make-up Artist

There are two basic methods for removing wrinkles temporarily. One technique consists of applying tiny tapes to the sides of the face to stretch up individual areas of the skin. The other technique is the use of a velour stretch band that smooths out the general contour of the face. These methods are used both in film and theatre and by the general public.

FACE-LIFT TAPES

Commercial face-lift tapes consist of two one-inch square pieces of clear surgical tape, attached to elastics that have eyelets and hooks in them for tension. You can make a simple version of this lift. You

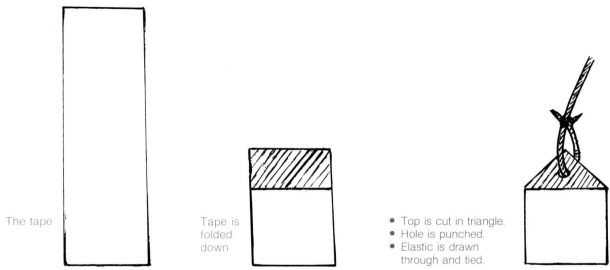

The tape

Tape is folded down

- Top is cut in triangle.
- Hole is punched.
- Elastic is drawn through and tied.

will need two pieces of round elastic cord, each approximately twelve inches long, and two pieces of clear surgical tape one inch wide and 3½ inches in length. Fold one end of the tape over three times to create a strong edge. Now cut the folded end into a triangle and punch a small hole in it. This will leave one inch of it still available to be used as the face-lift tapes. Push one end of the elastic through the hole and secure it with a tied knot.

1. Stand in front of the mirror and put your fingers in front of the ears. Pull back the skin until the area looks smooth and free of lines. Try the same thing at the neck area and the eye area. Wherever you decide to lift, that is the area where you will place the tapes. You may use one or more sets, but the usual place to put the tapes is in front of the ears to smooth out nose-to-mouth lines and lift the jowls.

2. The tapes are applied before the face is made-up. The areas where the tapes are to be placed must be dry and oil free. These areas should be cleansed with rubbing alcohol.

3. Place the adhesive side against the skin in any of these areas:

    A. In front of the ears.

    B. Past the outer corner of the eyes.

    C. Below and behind the ears.

    Press the tapes on firmly and rub gently for ten seconds to assure good contact.

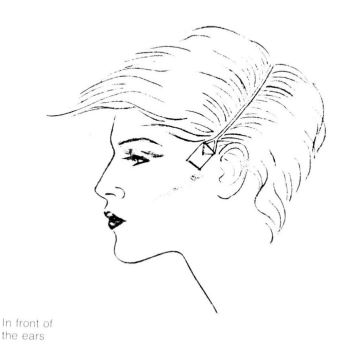

In front of
the ears

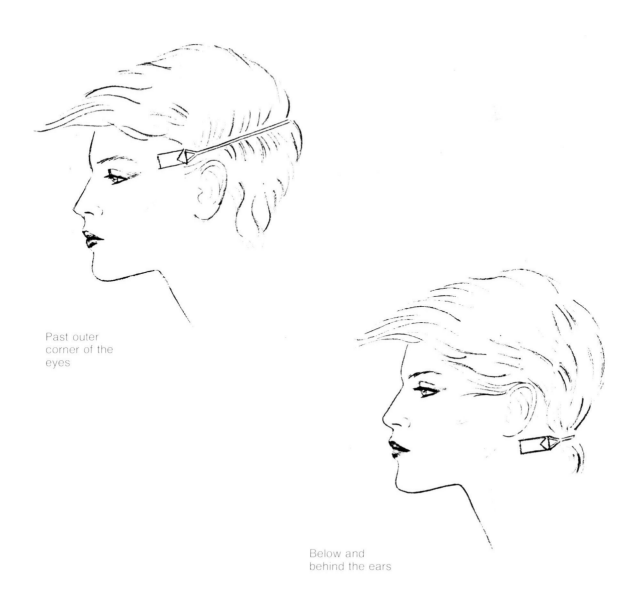

Past outer
corner of the
eyes

Below and
behind the ears

4. Separate the hair in back and comb the front part forward. Draw the elastics up across the back and top of the head, pulling the skin up smoothly but not so taut as to cause creases in the skin. Tie the ends of the elastics together. Use a bobby pin to keep the elastics in place. The hair is then combed back to conceal the elastic.

5. For the neck area you may draw the elastics up above the neckline into the separated hair and pin them into place securely. You must then dress the hair in a forward movement to cover the lifts. Little tendrils around the face are especially effective for this purpose. A short wig can be particularly useful too.

A fresh tape should be used each time. If you think that the tape needs extra security, you may use eyelash adhesive for extra hold. Pat on a small dot of adhesive to the lift area and let it dry before you apply the tapes.

THE FACE-LIFT BAND

The face-lift band is a two inch wide band of elasticized velour which, when properly worn, instantly smooths out the general contours of the face. When adjusted in place it firms the facial muscles and takes up the slack in the contours of the face. This technique of smoothing out facial lines is very popular with the famous actresses of the stage and screen. The commercially available band is adjustable and fits any head size. You may make your own version with an elastic velour band that is 2 inches wide and 16 to 18 inches long, depending on the size of the head. Possibly you can find this type of material at a fabric center. It is best to first make the band long enough to be worn comfortably. Test by pinning the ends together securely with safety pins. If it feels right, sew the ends together.

Now use the band as follows:

1. Draw the band down over the head to the neck. The velour side is inside against the head. The velour keeps the band from sliding.

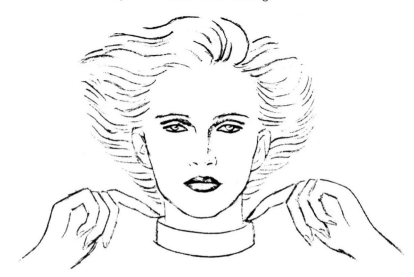

2. Grasp the upper edge of the band by the thumb and fingers and draw it upward against the face. The band must touch the face with tension constantly, as this is what draws the muscles upward.

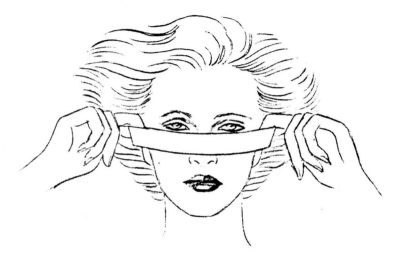

3. Bring the band against the forehead and draw it up approximately one to two inches beyond the hairline. Tilt the head backward to help the band adjust itself and release the earlobes. Straighten the head again and release the ears without lifting the beauty band.

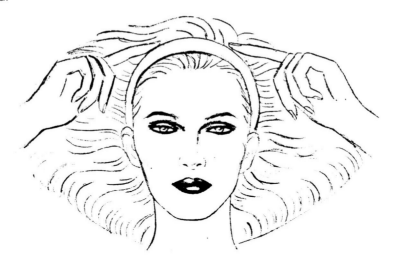

4. The hair is now combed into place. If the hair is long enough, at least shoulder length, it will merely appear as if the client were wearing a head band. If the hair is short, it may be necessary to conceal the band with a wig, scarf, bandeau or turban.

Section 2

Fashion, Film and Theatre

Chapter 7

Choosing Make-up for Various Media

Choosing the correct make-up for the individual model and situation is of the utmost importance. Much of course depends on the taste and choice of the make-up artist. Think of yourself as an artist about to paint a portrait. You look at the blank canvas which you have so carefully prepared. The first decision you must make is what the background color is to be. Once this is decided, you begin to apply a primary layer of paint which will give the painting its basic texture and tone. The same procedure is used when doing a creative make-up. Think of the skin's surface as the canvas and the features as the picture. It is only in this way that you can put your assignment in its proper perspective. Once you have grasped your patron's personality type and the situation for which she is being made-up, it is essential to free yourself from any inhibiting thoughts and think only of the portrait to be designed. As when painting a portrait, you will start to prime the canvas. The make-up base is your foundation and your object is to smooth the texture and even out the tone of the skin.

There are many types of make-up foundations ranging from translucent to those of great opacity that afford very heavy coverage. Three of the more popular bases are:

> **Fluid make-up:** Good for general use, it gives good coverage and is easy to apply. It can be made to have a matte finish by dusting it with a translucent powder.

> **Cream make-up:** (Stick or jar) A heavier type of make-up base, it is somewhat oily and can be powdered for lasting make-up. It provides excellent coverage and should be powdered for a matte-finish.

> **Cake make-up:** This base is applied with a damp sponge. Creating a completely matte finish, it provides top coverage and is not powdered.

CHOOSING COSMETICS FOR EVERYDAY USE

Choosing make-up bases

The most popularly used foundation is the fluid make-up. It is an emulsion type which is often a water-based make-up with a small percentage of oils. This type of make-up base can be used most successfully on a majority of skin types. The make-up artist should match the make-up base to the skin tone on the neck or jawline area. This is so there will be no line of demarcation where the make-up blends away.

Where there is an unwanted undertone to the skin coloring such as ruddiness, use a green tinted underbase. If the skin is particularly sallow, use a mauve underbase as a neutralizer.

For the older woman whose skin may have lost much of its youthful color it is best to warm the skin with a peachy make-up base rather than to match the paleness of the complexion.

Choosing eye-shadows

Eye-shadow colors were originally used to accentuate the color of the eye itself and people chose shadows which would harmonize with the color of the eye or would intensify the color through contrast. Although this is still done, today eye-shadow is used in a more sophisticated manner. Eye color is used as a costume accessory, picking up a color note from the dress, accessories or jewelry.

When choosing color to harmonize with the eye color, you might use this general guide...

EYE COLOR	EYE-SHADOW	SHADER	HIGHLIGHTER
Blue, Blue-grey	Blue, violet, turquoise, grey, plum	Charcoal, navy, purple, black	Pink, white, lilac, ivory
Green, Hazel, Light brown	Turquoise, apricot, green, cinnamon, taupe, peach	Brown, sienna, forest green, umber	Ivory, beige, yellow, peach
Dark brown, Black	Teal, apricot, turquoise, taupe, green, blue	Brown, black, charcoal, navy	Beige, ivory, yellow, pink

There are no hard and fast rules but you should be careful not to use a color that clashes with the general make-up or with the colors of the ensemble. Bright colors are usually best left for evening make-up.

Choosing the right lipstick

Your choice of a lipstick should primarily complement the skin and hair coloring and secondly coordinate with the costume colors.

As a general guide, you may follow this chart keyed to the hair color...

HAIR SHADE	LIPSTICK
Blonde, Grey, White	Pink, rose, lilac, peach, mocha, tawny
Golden blonde, Auburn, Titian	Russet, persimmon, coral, pink, orange-red, tawny, bronze, copper
Light Brown	Rose, clear red, tawny, lilac, coral
Dark brown, Black	Deep red, wine, berry colors, earth tones, bronze, plum

If the costume is a strong, definite color, such as purple, orange or red, coordinating the lipstick with the costume takes precedence over any other consideration.

Choosing a blush

It is not necessary to match the blush (accent rouge) to the lipstick but it should be in the same "cool" or "warm" color category. By this we mean, for example, that a coral lipstick may be worn with a bronze blush or a lilac lipstick may be worn with a pink blush. Use this chart as a guide to decide the warmth or coolness of a color. Cool colors are those with a blue undertone. Warm colors are earth toned or have a yellow undertone.

THE RED SCALE

COOL (Blue)—————CLEAR RED—————(Yellow) WARM

Blue-Red	Orange-Red
Lilac	Coral
Pink	Russet
Wine	Tawny
Raspberry	Bronze
Raisin	Peach
Mauve	Apricot
Fuschia	Mocha

MAKE-UP FOR COLOR PHOTOGRAPHY

Under ordinary situations in a fashion photography session the artist is not faced with any difficult decisions. No special techniques or adjustments are necessary and make-up can be applied in the same manner as for personal appearances. This is due to the super sensitivity of today's film to the full color spectrum and to the photographer's ability to vary color during the developing and printing processes; it is only necessary for the artist to handle colors with good taste. In other words, the colors you see are the colors you will get.

Make-up base

The first choice of a make-up base among fashion make-up artists is a lightly textured emulsion (water based) fluid base. One with enough coverage that is called for and one that spreads easily. The base must be matched to the neck area or, if changed for any reason, should be brought down onto the neck area. This is most important in color photography and, in fact, it is a good idea to always bring the color down onto the neck as the film can sometimes show a difference that the eye cannot discern.

Eye-shadows, blush and lipstick

Colors are chosen according to taste, taking into consideration wardrobe and background colors. Highly frosted eye-shadows and frosted lip gloss are best not used.

MAKE-UP FOR BLACK AND WHITE PHOTOGRAPHY

Black and white film does not register color as the eye sees it. The film registers everything on a grey scale from white to black with all tones in between registering as a shade of grey. Much depends upon the lighting conditions as to whether the colors will print light or dark. This is why when working with a photographer who is new to you it is best to check with him on his lighting setup before the actual shooting commences.

Make-up bases

Fluid make-up again is the primary choice but exact color choice is not as important. It is still best to choose the make-up by matching the skin on the neck area. On a very dark or black skin, it is sometimes useful to lighten the skin one or two shades so that the contouring and shading shows up to better advantage. Much depends on the lighting.

Eye-shadows

It is not necessary to concern yourself with the color of eye-shadows as everything registers in shades of grey. It is very difficult to judge what a blue shadow will look like or the shade of pink blush. It is, therefore, best to use only contouring and highlighting for the eyes utilizing browns, taupes, charcoal and black for shading and ivory, beige or white for highlighting.

Blush

In black and white photography, color is not used on the cheeks but rather the cheek bones are delineated with contouring and highlighting.

Use mocha, tawny or brownish shading rouge for the contouring in the cheek hollows (if desired). The height of the cheek bones may be highlighted merely with an extra sweep of the light translucent powder.

Lipstick

Use rose, tawny, coral, red or deep red tones depending on how dark you wish the lips to look. For example, a rose or coral lipstick will register as a middle grey, while a burgundy color will register very dark, as will a dark red.

SPECIAL HINTS FOR PHOTOGRAPHY

- A matte finish to the skin will photograph better than a shiny finish. You should remember to powder well.

- Frosted shadows may be used when called for but often photograph white. Use these shadows carefully. They also emphasize eye lines.

- A nonfrosted lip stick or lip gloss will be less likely to emphasize unwanted lines in the lips than a frosted lip product.

- For a beach or swimming scene a cream make-up may be best to use as it has sheen and will shed water.

- Many photographers use an instant photo to check their lighting. Ask to see the picture so that you can check your make-up.

- After you finish the make-up in the dressing room check the make-up again under the photographer's lights.

- If you have not worked with the photographer before, ask him if the contouring, lip gloss and blush are correct for his particular lighting. The photographer may sometimes want a little stronger or softer application.

- Keep a powder puff, blush and lipstick on the set ready for touch-ups.

MAKE-UP FOR COLOR FILM

Make-up application for movie film is very similar to that for print photography. As with color photography, the make-up foundation must be very close to the individual's skin coloring. The base should match the neck area, but if this is not the best choice due to the situation or characterization at hand, the make-up must be brought down onto the neck area.

Do not forget, in this case, to match and color all exposed skin on the hands and body. For the face, a cream base with light texture or cake make-up, if desired, is usually used. Make-up must be perfectly applied and kept natural looking for the searching eye of the camera. For hands and body you may wish to use cake make-up as it will have less of a tendency to rub off.

Special hints

- Follow the rules for color print photography.

- Make sure to view the test filming that is usually done for wardrobe and hair. Make-up will be an important part of the test and you can determine if any changes need to be made before the actual filming of the movie starts.

MAKE-UP FOR TELEVISION

Make-up base

The type of make-up base to use is either the cream or cake type. Cream make-up may be somewhat easier to blend but cake make-up may be preferable for an oily skin. The make-up should be applied in a very light film and kept very natural looking. Generally, the base should be of a beige or warm beige tone.

Theatrical make-up companies make a special series of bases for television and they are probably the safest for the beginner to use. For example, if the make-up runs in a series of from TV 1 to TV 10, a woman could use TV 4 or 5 depending on her coloring and a man would use TV 6 to 8. Base color is usually a little deeper than the natural coloring for the very light skinned so it should be brought down to the neck area also. Be sure not to forget to cover the hands and shoulders if necessary. For black skin a shade of base that complements and blends with the complexion is all that is needed.

Shading and highlighting

All corrective work can be accomplished with the same series. Shading may be accomplished with a base 2 to 4 shades deeper than the original base and highlighting with a base 3 to 4 shades lighter. TV cameras differ as does the lighting, from studio to studio, so that when you become familiar with the individual studio setup you can experiment with other bases and other techniques.

Eye-shadow

It is best to use soft muted colors for television and to avoid frosts. So far as color is concerned, "when in doubt, leave it out." Colors such as taupes, mushroom and grey browns are safe particularly for contouring. Skin tone itself can be the highlighting.

Blush and lipstick

Some TV cameras exaggerate red tones so it is safest to use tones of tawny, coral or soft pink. Beware of using too much cheek blush. It often looks stronger to the camera than to the naked eye. **For men,** an amber or tawny blush may be skillfully applied, and buffed to a very natural look. No lipstick is ordinarily used for men. If the natural lips are very red they may be toned down by applying a little base over them.

Special hints for television make-up

- Make-up should have a matte finish for television.

- It is best not to use any frosted make-up products for television as it may have unwanted reflective properties.

- Colors often seem a little brighter to the camera particularly red shades, so ask to view your client on camera before shooting starts. This can be accomplished by going into the control room and seeing the colors correctly on a screen.

- Application of the shading before the general base will give a more natural look to the contouring.

MAKE-UP FOR THE STAGE

There are many variables in making-up someone for the stage. For one thing it is important to take into consideration the size of the theatre. There is the *Intimate* theatre with up to 100 seats, the *Mid-Ranged* theatre with up to 300 seats and the *Long-Ranged* theatre with a seating capacity of 300 or more. In a very small theatre make-up must be put on with discretion and look natural at fairly close range. In larger theatres it is often necessary to exaggerate the make-up somewhat in order to better project the features and the character.

Lighting

The lighting used on stage will affect the appearance of the make-up colors. Lighting designers will often use various "gels" over the lights to obtain certain color effects and the make-up artist must be prepared to adjust the make-up application accordingly.

The popular amber gels are quite soft and flattering to most make-ups. If they are deep, however, they may fade the lipstick and rouge slightly, calling for make-up somewhat more intense. Red gels will fade and sometimes completely cancel out red shades even more so. Blue lights will add violet to reds in make-up and even cause them to appear black. Green obviously will add its own cast to the skin and make lipsticks appear brownish.

Make-up bases

The bases used for stage are usually of the cream or cake type. Undertones as a general rule are in the warm or red-orange category. For men, bronze or suntanned tones are used. Needless to say, much depends on the character the actor or actress has to portray. Obviously a young man of twenty playing a robust or outdoor type will have a much different coloring than one playing a studious or bookish type. In general, the make-up base is somewhat deeper than the natural skin tone.

Eye-shadow

Shading, contouring and highlighting are essential for the stage. Eyes should be well defined with liner; this includes the eyes of men but with much more subtlety. Bright shades of eye-shadow are best kept for roles that call for that type of look. Avoid highly frosted eye-shadows.

Blush and lipstick

Blush and lipstick are chosen in the regular manner to coordinate with the general make-up, costume, or character portrayed.

Special hints for stage make-up

For a realistic contouring of the face do shading and highlighting with creams before the base is applied. After powdering, the contouring can be reemphasized with powdered shaders and highlighters. This type of make-up will stand up for a longer period of time under the lights.

Chapter 8

Corrective Make-up Using the Chiaroscuro Technique

Chiaroscuro make-up is ideal from every standpoint of beauty. Because it utilizes earth tones it can look very natural. Applied in a stronger manner it can look very high fashion. It is also ideal for both black and white and color photography.

DETERMINING PROPER COLOR SCHEME FOR PHOTOGRAPHING CHIAROSCURO

Under ideal lighting conditions color film will register a make-up just as the eye does. Black and white film, on the other hand, sees everything in varying shades of grey, ranging in extremes from white to black. Since bright or light colors do not necessarily register on film with the same intensity that the eye perceives them, it is best not to use them. Blue eye-shadows, for example, though outstanding in color, may register as non-existant in the photo. On the other hand, red rouge may photograph dark and therefore create a shadow on the cheek where we would prefer a highlight. From this example, you can see that it is somewhat more sensible to use a scale of colors from which you can easily determine the shade of grey that will register on film.

CHOOSING MAKE-UP TONES

The Chiaroscuro make-up utilizes earth tones of cosmetics in various degrees of depth. Choose a make-up base with a beige undertone and eye-shadows in taupes and browns or greys and blacks. Use shading rouges with a mocha or tawny base, and lipsticks in amber rose, cafe or sienna. Eye crayons can be deep brown, black and charcoal. Mascara should be black or brown-black. If the skin is tan to black you may wish to use rouges and lipsticks in raisin, plum or wine in order to show up as a better contrast. Start out with earth tones and you can vary your choices as you get more familiar with the technique.

CHOOSING COLOR INTENSITY

In choosing the depth of the intensity of color or its value (light to dark) keep in mind the color's contrast with the skin color. A deeply tan, brown or dark brown skin color will need darker contouring than a fair or pale skin will need. The same fair skin will need a much lighter highlight for contrast than will a dark skin. Should you wish to do a make-up that is somewhat livelier in color, you may use a brighter lipstick in the medium red or coral tone, and pink or coral blusher on the fullness of the cheeks. The medium red lipstick will probably photograph as a middle grey tone and the rouge, if light, will not register deep enough on black and white film to effect it. This may be an ideal solution if the photographer is shooting in both color and black and white film.

APPLICATION OF CHIAROSCURO MAKE-UP

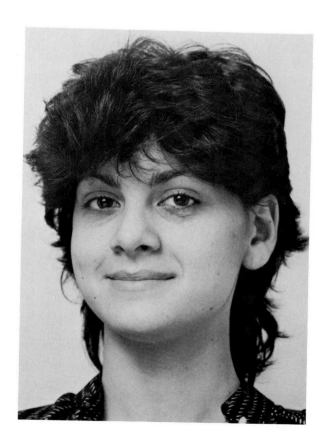

Photo 1
In this photo the model, Barbara, is shown without make-up, in her usual hairstyle.

Photo 2
Barbara's hair is pulled back and held with a head band. The skin is cleansed and toned, and a light moisturizer is applied. Her well-shaped brows need no correcting.

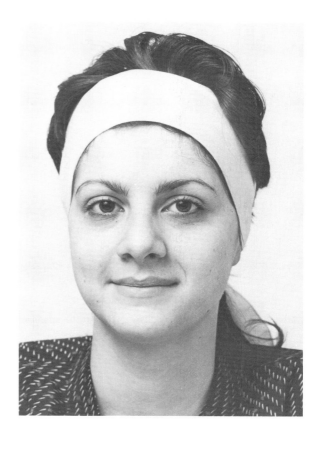

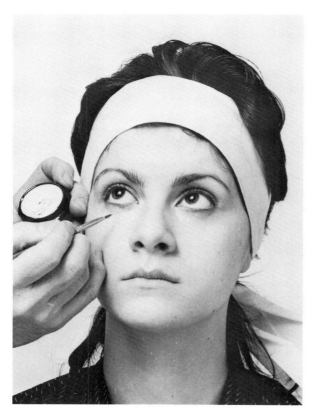

Photo 3
A concealer is brushed onto the under-eye area. It is then blended with the fingertips or a sponge if you prefer. It is also applied to the inner and outer corners of the eye area to conceal slight discolorations and applied to any blemishes.

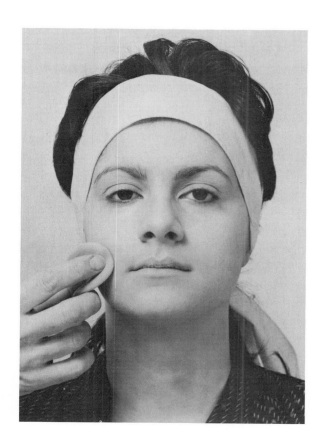

Photo 4
A fluid make-up base is dotted all over the face with the fingertips and then blended with a latex sponge. The base color was chosen by matching the skin tone on the neck area. Therefore it is only necessary to bring the make-up just under the jawline area.

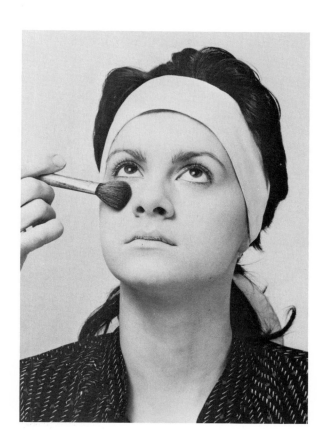

Photo 5
A translucent powder is brushed over the entire face, including the eyelids. This is to add a matte finish and help set the make-up. For a more lasting matte finish, the powder can be pressed on with a velour puff rather than applied with a brush.

Photo 6

An ivory matte eye-shadow was applied to the entire eyelid area. This evens out the skin tone and acts as a base for the contouring shadow that will be used. When working on the upper eyelid the index finger is placed on the browbone and the skin drawn taut in an oblique manner. This allows the product to be brushed on more evenly.

Here a beige-brown matte shadow is being applied to the center or depth area of the lid. Color is concentrated on the outer part to add more dramatic depth. During application the model's eyes are kept closed and the skin held taut.

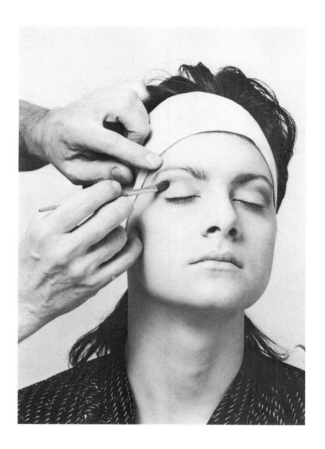

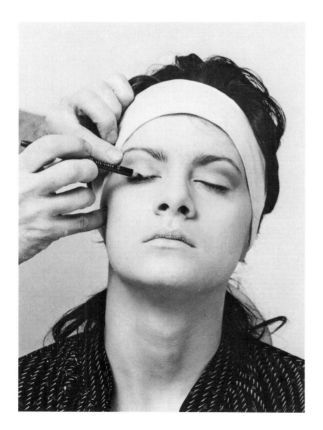

Photo 7

To outline the eyes, a dark brown lining pencil is used. Starting near the inner eye corner a fine line is drawn at the base of the lashes widening slightly as it reaches the outer corner of the eye.

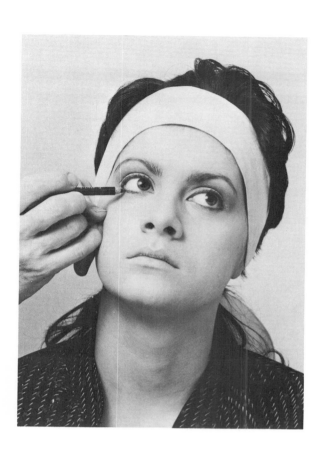

Photo 8

With the same pencil a line is drawn on the lower lid at the base of the lashes. The line starts about one third of the way out from the inner corner and joins the liner on the upper lid at the outer corner of the eye. The lower liner is then softened by blending it gently with the tip of a sponge shadow applicator.

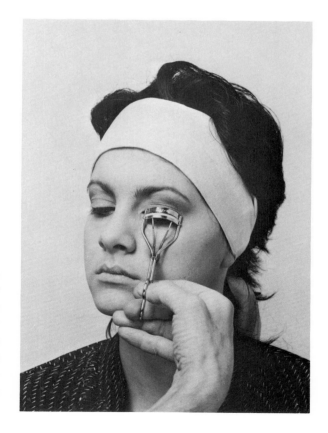

Photo 9

An eyelash curler is now used to gently curl the lashes upward. The hand holding the curler rests against the chin for security while the curler closes carefully on the lashes. The curler relaxes and closes five or six times at the base of the lashes and then is moved toward the tips of the lashes. The closing and relaxing movement is repeated. Curling the lashes is always done before mascara is applied.

Photo 10

Mascara is now applied to the bottom lashes. Barbara has lovely long lashes but the bottom lashes are fairly light and need a careful application of mascara. Again resting the small finger of the hand against the face for security, the tip of the mascara wand is brushed back and forth coating lashes with mascara. The mascara wand is then held horizontally and the lashes are separated.

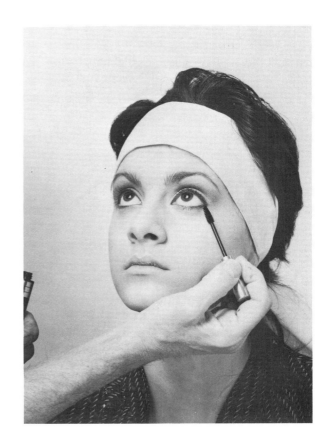

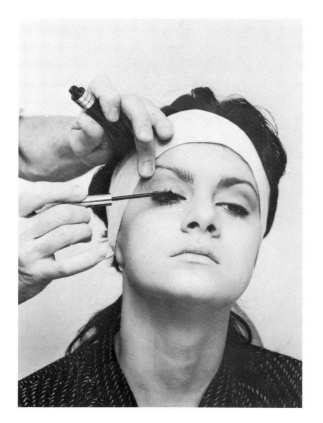

Photo 11

When mascara is applied to the top lashes the model looks down while the lid is held taut. The mascara is first brushed on the top of the lashes and then brushed on from underneath. To build up the thickness of the lashes the mascara is allowed to dry, separated with a brush or mascara comb and then another application of mascara is applied.

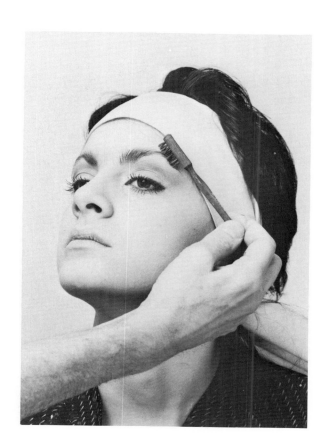

Photo 12
A brow brush is used to brush the brows upward and outward. A spray of hair spray or lacquer on the brush will help hold the hairs in place.

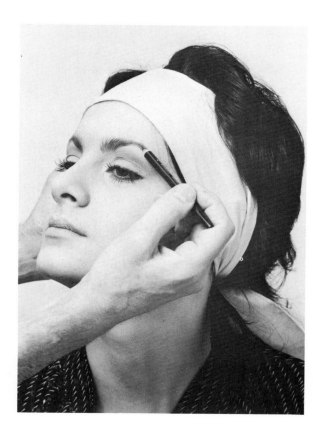

Photo 13
Fill in the brow where needed using a well sharpened dark brown eyebrow pencil. Be sure to use small pencil strokes.

Photo 14

Use a tawny or mocha shade of rouge to contour the cheeks. The model draws her cheeks in to delineate the cheek bones. The shading rouge is brushed on in the hollow of the cheek in a line approximately under the outer corner of the eye and continues up toward the top of the ear.

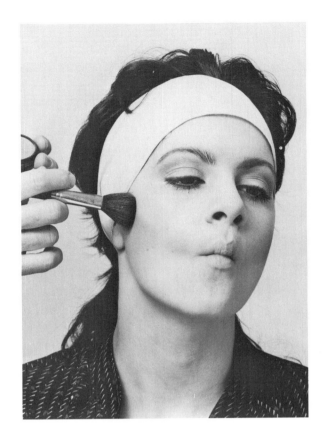

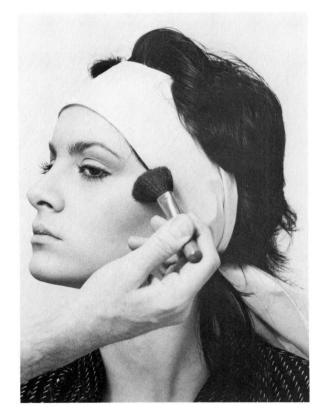

Photo 15

The rouge is brushed up onto the fullness of the cheeks and fades away at the height of the cheek bone. The strength of the color remains at the hollow of the cheek bone. If more shading is desired, a fawn or beige-brown rouge or shader can be applied to the hollow. This must be done very lightly. A dry puff of cotton may be delicately rubbed over the edges to blend the shades. A translucent powder is then fluffed on the entire area if needed to soften the effect.

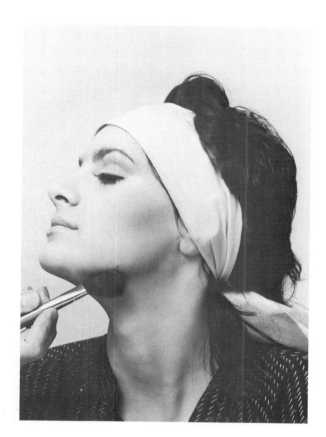

Photo 16
The jawline is contoured by applying a fawn or tawny shading rouge starting under one ear and continuing directly under the edge of the jawline to the other ear.

Photo 17

To sculpture the nose we use the beige-brown shader applied with a small shading brush. We start a little above eye level down toward the tip of the nose. A quarter of an inch area is left clear, down the center of the nose. Edges are blended very carefully leaving no apparent lines of demarcation. This technique is excellent for black and white photography and for evening make-up.

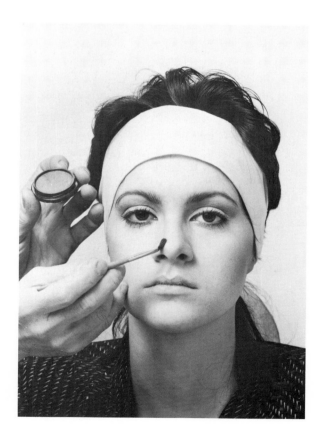

Photo 18
Lips are outlined and then filled in with lip color.
A ruddy brown lip liner is used and the lip color is
a middle tone russet shade of lipstick. Lip gloss
may be used if desired but very lightly. Usually a
creamy lipstick provides sufficient shine.

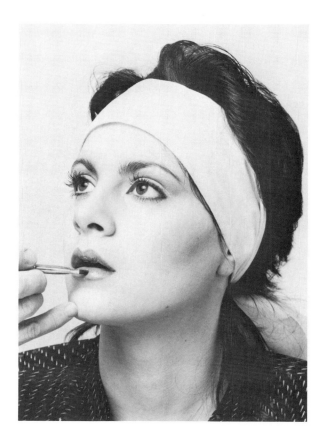

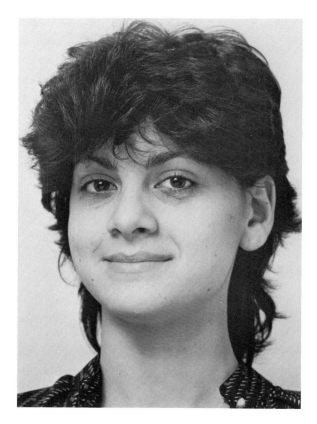

Photo 19
Here is Barbara before the transformation. In
the finished photos you can see how a
corrective make-up can diminish facial flaws
and emphasize the good features.

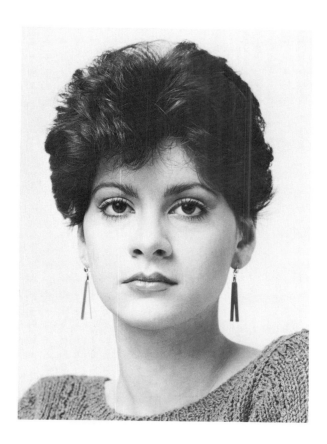

Photo 20
Here is the finished make-up with the hair arranged in a somewhat more sophisticated style.

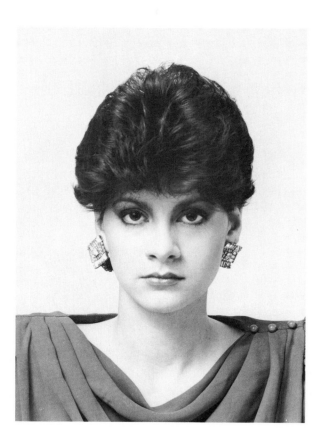

Photo 21
In this photo the features have been contoured in deeper shades for extra definition. Eye make-up is also more exaggerated for that high fashion look.

Chapter 9

Make-up for the Black Woman

Make-up for the Black woman is not that much different than make-up for the Caucasian woman. The application of make-up is very similar but there are a few characteristics that may be taken into consideration when making-up a Black woman.

SPECIAL CONSIDERATIONS

1. There is a very large range of skin color among Blacks ranging from a pale tan to a dark brown or almost black coloring. Undertones may be yellow, copper or even blue. It is important to choose a foundation that matches or blends well with the natural skin tones. Often the skin on the neck is darker than the face, so match the foundation to the skin tones of the face.

2. On the darker skin it is often better to highlight an area rather than to rely on shading. For example, one could highlight the height of the cheek bone and let the natural skin tone in the cheek hollow be its own shading by contrast.

3. The nose may be somewhat broad and may need to be sculptured with shading. This is particularly so when being photographed since front lighting has a tendency to flatten the features.

4. Full lips are often well in balance with the rest of the features. When lips are overly full it is best to stay away from bright, light and frosted lipsticks. Earth tones are safest.

SKIN PREPARATION

After the make-up was removed with cleanser, an astringent for oily skin was applied. The next step was a touch of moisturizer around the eyes, lips, and throat, with any excess being blotted off with a tissue.

APPLICATION OF MAKE-UP

A base is chosen that is close to the skin coloring of the face. For black and white photography it is sometimes necessary to use a foundation slightly lighter than the natural skin coloring. This is so shading and contouring will show up better on film. For stage lighting, foundation can be slightly darker than the natural skin tone. Much depends on the lighting and how much it washes out the natural coloring. The make-up base is applied with a sponge and blended over the entire face, down the jawline and onto the neck area. Occasionally, make-up may give the dark skin an ashen tone. This may be caused by the titanium dioxide that is added to some bases to give opacity to the product. If this ashiness does occur, add some red or orange cream make-up to the base to neutralize the unwanted tone.

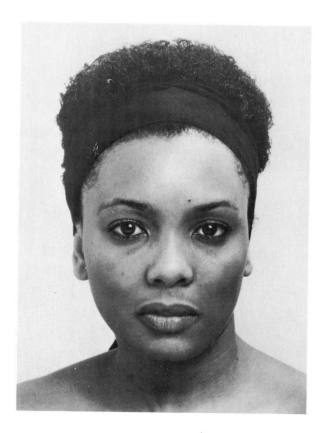

Photo 1
Here we see our model with no make-up at all. Her lovely oval face and well-balanced features will need only a good basic application of corrective make-up to make the most of her beauty potential.

Photo 2
A concealer is applied to the under-eye area to lighten dark shadows. If there is a puff under the eyes put the cover-up on the dark area and not on the puff itself. Blend and feather the concealer. If the concealer is very much lighter than the skin tone it may be preferable to apply it before the base, on the under-eye area.

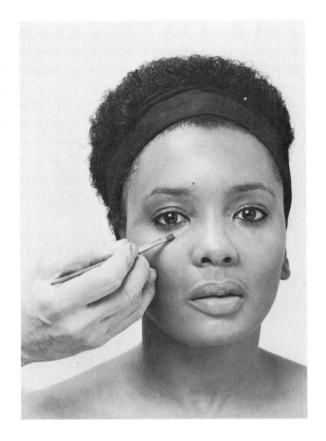

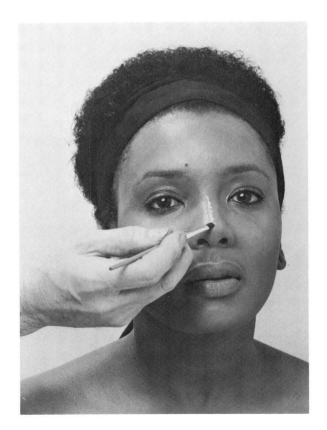

Photo 3
A thin line of the concealer, used as a highlighter, is then applied to the center of the nose. It can be applied to the naso-labial fold to lighten it if necessary.

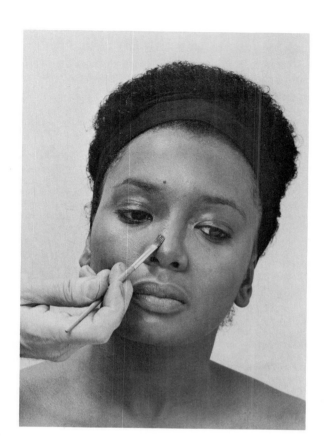

Photo 4
A shading cream in brown, or even black if the skin is very dark, may be brushed down the sides of the nose for a sculpturing effect. Other features that may be diminished might be a too-pointed chin, jowls or a double chin. If a shading powder rather than a cream is to be used for sculpturing, it is applied after powdering the face.

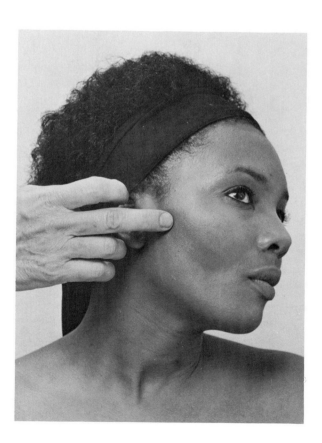

Photo 5
The shading cream is stroked on in the hollow of the cheek, in a line starting under the outer corner of the eye and runs up toward the top of the ear. Blend with the finger tips or a sponge.

Photo 6
Three dots of cream rouge are applied to the height of the cheek bone. Since we decided to use colors on the blue side of the red scale, the blush is fuschia tone and will give the cheeks a nice color accent.

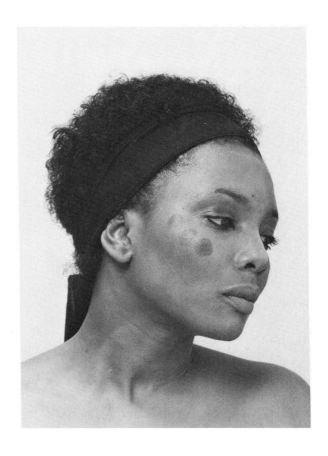

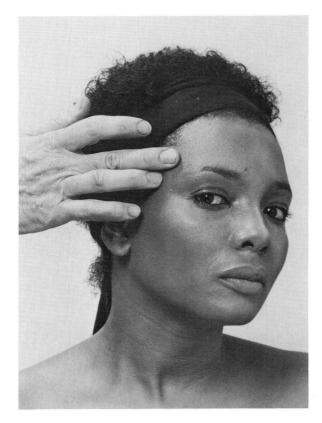

Photo 7
The blush is blended down into the shading in the cheek hollow and up to the temporal area. The edges are well feathered allowing no lines of demarcation. The face and neck are powdered down with a translucent powder to set the make-up.

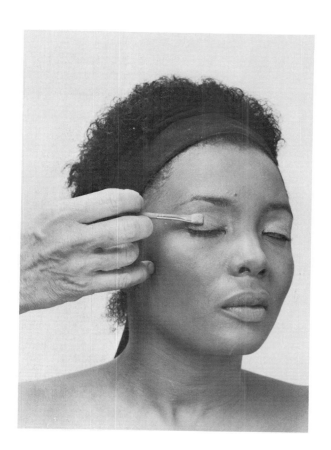

Photo 8

A teal powdered eye-shadow, brushed on the eyelid, will accentuate the beauty of the eyes and coordinate with the costume color. If desired, the eye-shadow may be wrapped around the outer third of the bottom lid acting as a frame to the eyes.

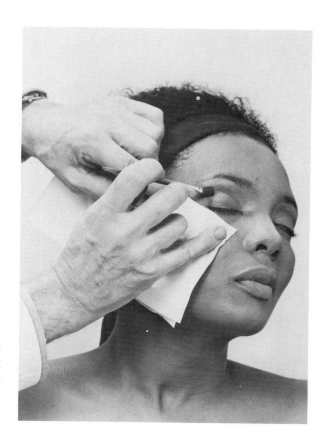

Photo 9

A dark powdered shadow is brushed on the center or depth area of the eye for contour. It may be dark brown, navy or black. A tissue is held against the cheek to catch any flaking from the eye-shadow.

Photo 10
A black cake eye-liner is used on the top lid. The eyelid is held upward so that the liner can be painted on in a smooth even line right down at the base of the lashes. A black crayon may be used instead, but cake eye-liner will hold up better particularly for stage make-up. This is true for all make-ups, not only for black women.

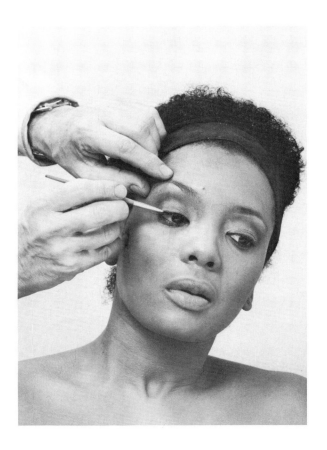

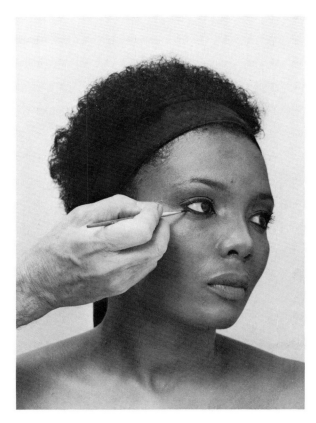

Photo 11
Starting about one third out from the inner eye corner black eye-liner is drawn on at the base of the lashes and meets the upper liner at the outer corner.

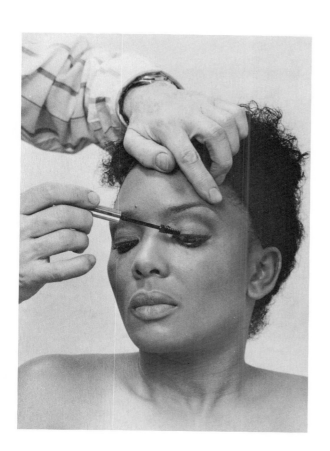

Photo 12
Black mascara is stroked on to the lower and upper eyelashes.

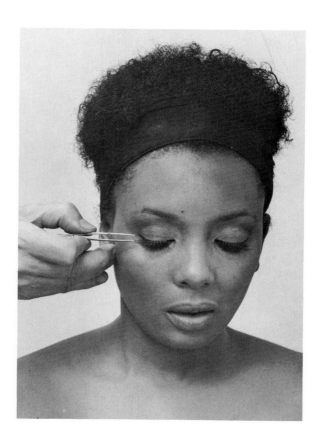

Photo 13
Black, spiky lashes on a strip are attached. These are applied directly at the base of the lashes. False lashes are not necessarily used for fashion but are very attractive on stage.

Photo 14
Eyebrows are filled in with a well-sharpened pencil. Little hair-like strokes are sketched on for a natural effect.

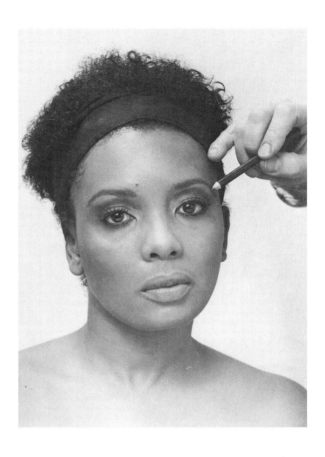

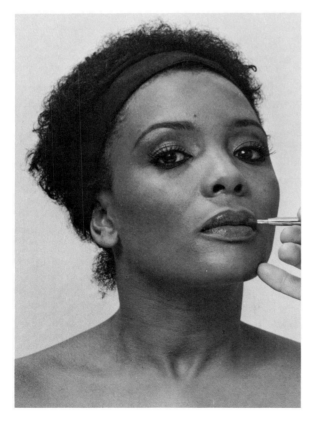

Photo 15
A raisin tinted lip color is brushed onto the lips. Sometimes the lower lip is of a lighter color than the top lip. This can be evened out in a number of ways. One way is to block out the lips before applying lip color, using a dark cover-stick. Powder over the cover-up and then apply the lip color. Another method is merely to use a darker shade of lip color on the lower lip than used on the upper lip. Be sure that they are in the same color category.

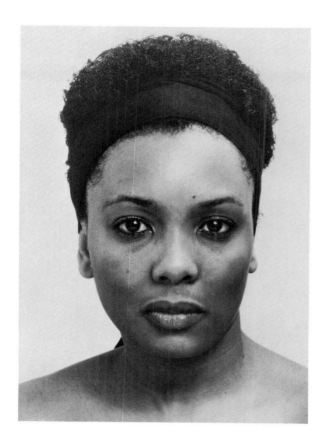

Photo 16
Looking back once more at our model before the make-up application clearly points up the importance of corrective make-up.

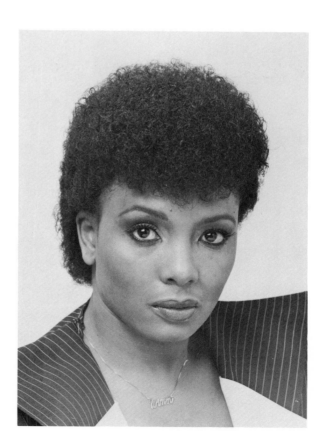

Photo 17
With make-up and hair completed, we see our model looking her best although not overly made-up.

Chapter 10

Make-up for the Oriental Woman

Make-up for the Oriental woman is both interesting and artistically satisfying. Because of the typically exotic features of the Oriental face, it lends itself to a variety of lovely make-up interpretations.

SPECIAL CONSIDERATIONS

Photograph 1 illustrates the characteristics of the Oriental face that should be kept in mind when applying make-up.

1. Facial shape is often broad with high cheek bones. Because of the width of the face, the cheek bones can appear to be flat.

2. The nose is short with a low bridge at the level of the eye area. The eyes are usually level with the facial surface. The epicanthic fold or eye fold covers the entire eyelid often reaching down as far as the upper eyelashes. As the fold draws the eye down at the inner corner it shapes the eye even more into an oblique or slanted contour.

3. The skin tone is on the beige side ranging from creamy ivory to sallow and olive variations. Skin texture is often seemingly poreless and quite smooth.

4. Eyebrows grow fairly straight with the hairs slanting downward. Eyelashes are very short and straight and also have a tendency to slant down.

The following pages illustrate make-up techniques which can be used to enhance the Oriental woman's naturally beautiful features.

APPLICATION OF MAKE-UP

Photo 1
In this first photograph our model is seen with very little make-up.

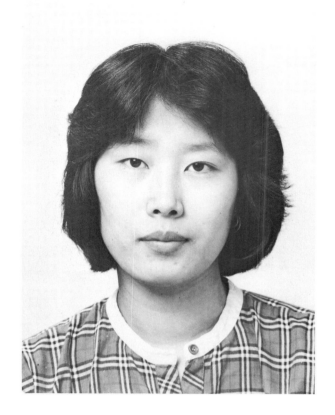

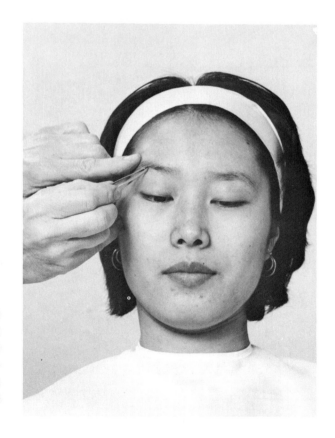

Photo 2
After the face is cleansed, the eyebrows are tweezed and reshaped. To give the brows an arch, the hairs are tweezed out from under the high point of the brow. Skin toner and moisturizer are applied. If the skin is very sallow a mauve tinted neutralizer may be patted on to counteract this undertone.

Photo 3
A creamy beige fluid make-up base is dotted all over the face.

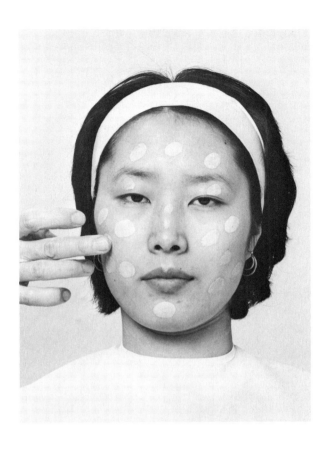

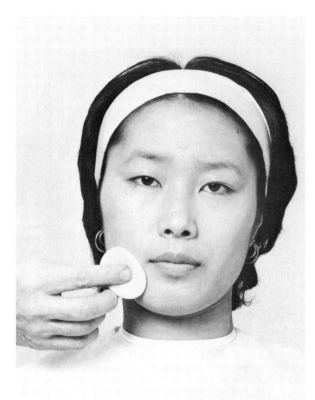

Photo 4
A sponge is used for application, including the eyelid area and the lips. The make-up is brought down under the jawline and blended away.

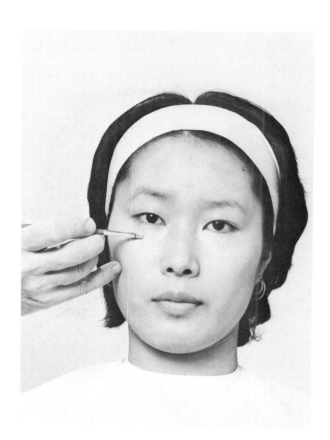

Photo 5
Concealer is applied to the under-eye area with a brush. It is then blended with the fingertips.

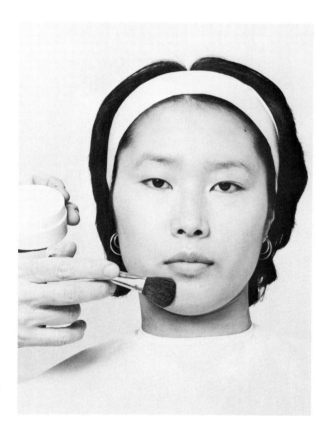

Photo 6
Translucent powder is brushed on to give the skin a smooth, matte finish.

Photo 7

A soft black eye-shadow is now applied to the upper eye area. The skin is held taut in an upward and outward manner to lift the eye fold off the eyelid. The eye-shadow is then brushed on in an almond shape starting just past the inner eye corner and rising upward gradually in a line past the outer eye corner.

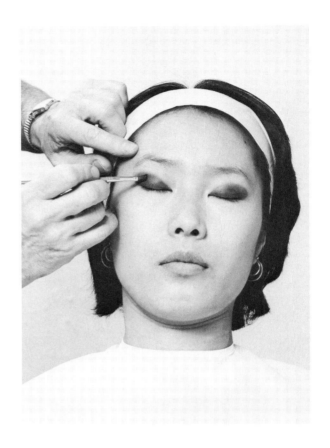

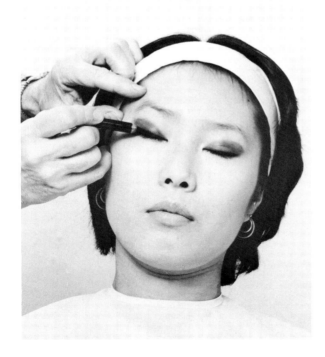

Photo 8

While the eyelid is lifted and held taut, liner is drawn in at the lash base with a black eye crayon starting very thin at the inner corner and becoming quite thick at the end. In order for the eye-liner to be seen at all when the eye is opened, the crayon is applied not only to the eyelid itself but thick enough so that it is drawn onto the fold also.

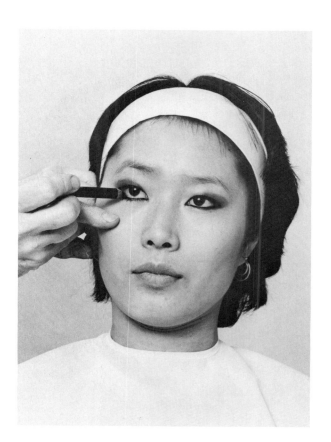

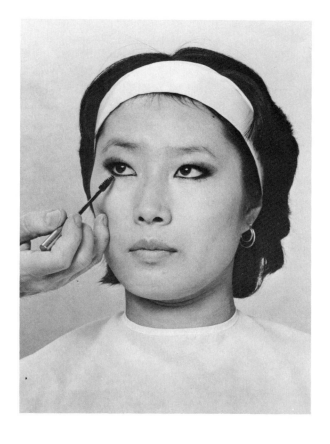

Photo 9
Liner is also applied to the lower lid area both at the base of the lashes and directly above to the rim of the lid.

Photo 10
Mascara is brushed into the lower lashes only. The small finger rests against the cheek to give the hand control. The mascara wand is wisked back and forth to deposit the mascara and then held horizontally to separate the lashes. Mascara is not applied to the upper lashes because of the intent to use false eyelashes. Our model's lashes are fairly short and straight and if mascara were applied they would appear as separate from the false lashes. Without mascara they will be less noticeable.

Photo 11

Short, curly artificial strip lashes are applied directly at the base of the real lashes. Lashes should start at least ¼ inch away from the inner corner of the eye.

Eyebrows are filled in by sketching in hair-like strokes with a very sharply pointed dark brown pencil. The entire brow is then softened with a dry eyebrow brush. If need be, a light application of powder will soften an obviously penciled in eyebrow.

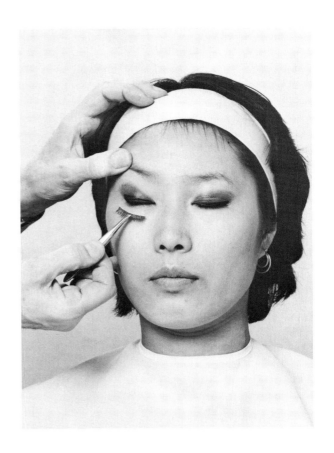

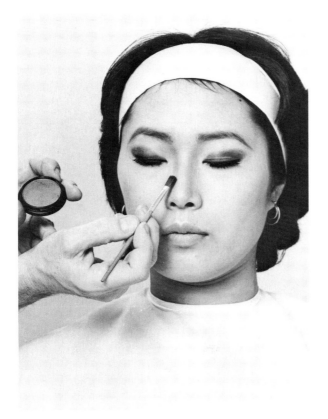

Photo 12

A faun colored shading rouge is applied with a flat brush to the sides of the nose. When sculpturing a short nose, the shader can be stroked on from the inner part of the eyebrow to the tip of nose. This should be done very lightly and blended well. A quarter inch space is left down the center of the nose. It cannot be emphasized enough that this technique though ideal for black and white photography and also for evening make-up might best be skipped for daytime make-up and color photography. In the latter, it may show up as a muddy or brownish smudge.

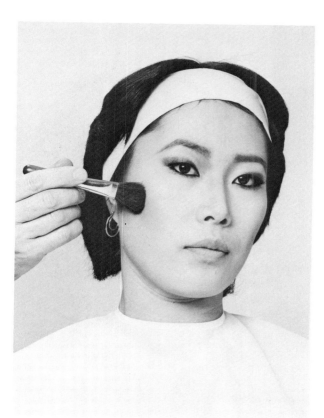

Photo 13
A mocha colored shading blush is brushed on. The model draws in her cheeks to delineate the cheek bones and the blusher is brushed on in the hollow of the cheeks and softly brushed up to but not onto the height of the cheek bones.

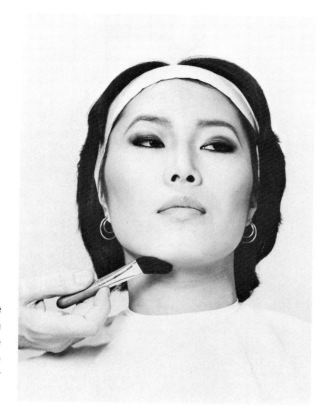

Photo 14
The faun blush is now brushed along the underside of the jawline. Starting from beneath the earlobe on one side and continued onto the other side of the jawline. This strengthens the jawline and reduces any sign of fullness under the chin.

Photo 15
The lips are first outlined with a lip pencil and then filled in with lip color.

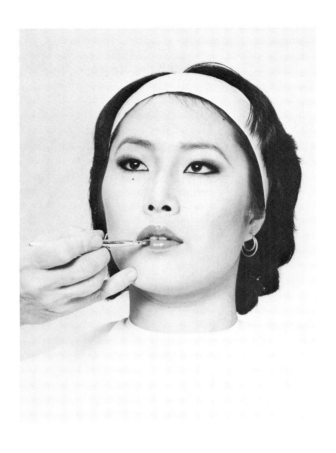

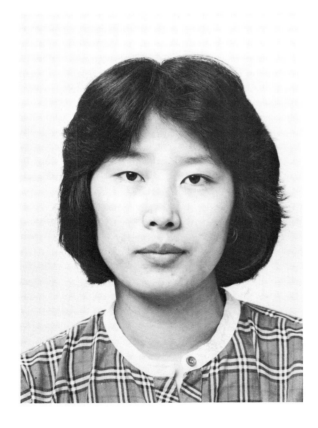

Photo 16
Looking at this picture and then at photo 17, you can clearly see that a simple application of relatively few cosmetics has made a world of difference in this Oriental beauty.

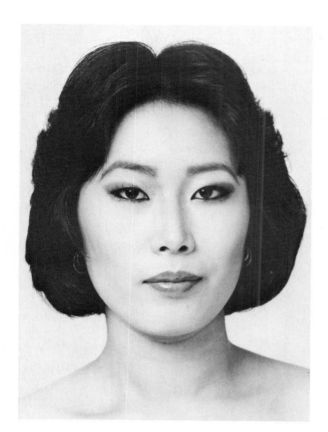

Photo 17

Here in the finished picture we see a softly elegant and fashionable make-up. Of course this is only one way to design a make-up for the Oriental woman. Use your imagination and vary your technique in applying eye make-up to obtain individual looks.

SPECIALIZED TECHNIQUE: THE ARTIFICIAL CREASE LINE

This is a slightly more complicated eye design which you may want to try. By emphasizing and even recreating the crease line you can dramatize the eyes to a great degree. The technique is also useful for any woman whose eye shape must be exaggerated, such as a stage actress, runway model or ballerina.

1. A deep shade of shadow such as brown, or charcoal is applied to the center portion or depth area of the eyelid. The shadow is blended very carefully. The edges must blend away without any apparent line of demarcation.

2. A brown or black cake eye-liner, weakened to transparency with extra water, is used to create a crease line. With a fine brush a line is drawn in lightly over the center portion of the depth area to give the impression of a natural crease line or eye fold.

BEFORE

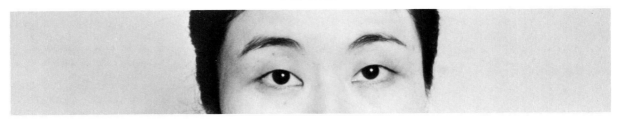

AFTER

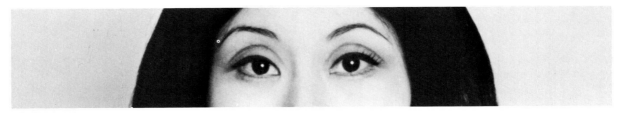

Chapter 11

Make-up for the Mature Woman

Make-up can make a woman look prettier, softer, more glamourous and yet make-up can also, if applied incorrectly, accentuate lines, harden the features and add age. There is no one way to apply make-up to the mature woman any more than there is only one way to make-up a young lady. One must take into consideration such things as the personality type, the lifestyle and the condition of the skin. If one can generalize for the mature woman it is safe to suggest a lighter touch to the make-up, softer colors, and matte eye-shadow and liner. The make-up foundation may be a water base, or if the skin is quite dry one could choose an oil base type. A light touch is always in order to avoid make-up collecting in facial lines, particularly face powder.

SPECIAL CONSIDERATIONS

Here is how to work with some typical facial problems associated with the mature woman:

1. Puffs under the eye are often a problem. A concealing cream to lighten the shadow immediately under the puff should be used. Apply the concealer with a thin, flat brush. If the puffs are prominent, pat on a slightly deeper base to the puffy areas only. The base combined with the concealer on the shadow underneath will have the effect of flattening out the puffs.

2. To eliminate dark under-eye shadows stretch the skin under the eyes and apply concealer with the finger tips. Remove all excess and powder very lightly. If the powder tends to exaggerate facial lines, it might be better not to use any.

3. An exaggerated naso-labial fold can also be a problem with the mature woman. To soften these nose to mouth lines apply concealer or highlighter inside the lines using a thin pointed brush. Pat to remove all excess.

4. If the skin is particularly dry or lined, use an emollient cream such as a night cream rather than a moisturizer. Apply before the base and blot it well with tissue.

5. A highlighter or concealer cream may be used to lighten dark pockets at the inner corner of the eye and also at the outer corners.

6. Very often the skin tone fades as a woman grows older. Do not attempt to match the skin color but rather use a peachy or somewhat pinker base color.

7. If the eyelid area is droopy or puffy do not attempt to do a standard contouring. Use muted shadows to diminish the area, such as grey-blue, hush-brown, and mocha. Apply a thin line of brighter color just above the lash line to add a dash of brightness to the eyes. Very fine, short false lashes can be a great beautifier for this type of eye.

APPLICATION OF MAKE-UP
(Including face-lift tape procedure)

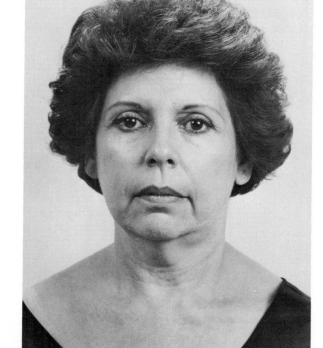

Photo 1

Our model is seen here with her regular make-up. She has a good complexion, well-defined features and good eye proportion. To be corrected are the lines at the outer corner of the lips and the slight droop at the outer corner of the eyelids. These defects cannot be successfully corrected with make-up so we will use face lift tapes to physically smooth the lines away.

Photo 2

A thorough cleansing, application of skin freshener and moisturizer prepared the skin for the make-up application. If the model has particularly dry skin, apply a light film of an emollient type cream. Blot off all excess cream.

A fluid make-up base is chosen in a color that blends into the neck area. If your base seems too heavy, you may add a few drops of water to thin it and perhaps a bit of moisturizer. The base is dotted all over the face and then blended in with a latex sponge. The base is brought down under the jawline and gradually blends away towards the neck.

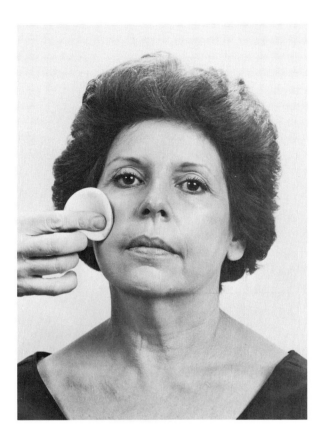

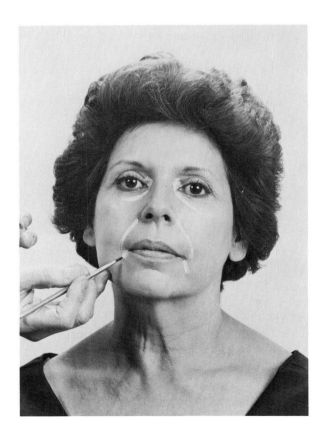

Photo 3

A brush is used to apply cover-up to the shadows on the under-eye area, the naso-labial fold and the lines at the outer corner of the lips.

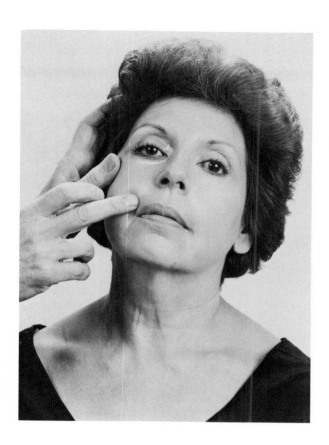

Photo 4
The cover-up is blended into the surrounding area and the edges feathered. This may be accomplished with the fingertips or a sponge.

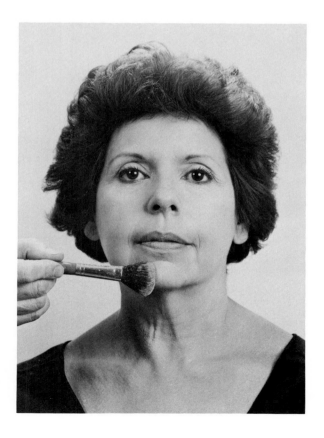

Photo 5
A translucent powder is applied to set the make-up and give it a soft matte finish. When using a powder brush, tap off the excess powder back into the powder container before using it. If a puff is used, first pick up the powder onto the puff and then fold the puff together working the powder into it. Now press the puff lightly but firmly against the skin working on the nose area, under the eyes, forehead and chin and cheeks. Do not rub the powder in but rather press it on. Excess can then be brushed off with the powder brush.

Photo 6

For eye color accent choose a color that has softness and brightness at the same time. Blue-grey, aqua and rose are all appropriate shades. Always avoid frosted shades if there is puffiness or any lined skin on the lid area.

The color accent is applied close to the lash line and blended up to the center area actually following the shape of the eye itself. In the photo a darker shadow is being applied to the outer portion of the eye fold to add depth to that area. A color such as plum, dark grey or faun is a good choice.

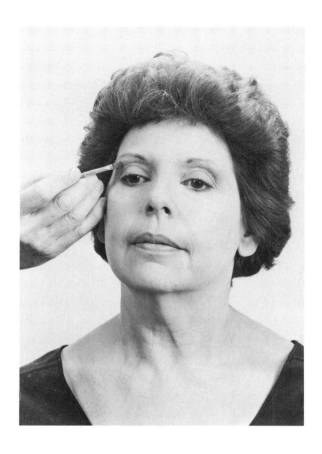

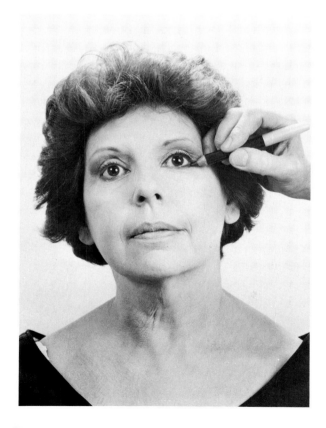

Photo 7

For lining the eyes a charcoal, dark brown or navy crayon may be used. Liner is first applied to the top lid from near the inner corner out to the outer corner. The lower liner starts at the center and meets the liner at the outer corner. The lower liner should be applied softer than the top liner or it should be gently smudged to soften.

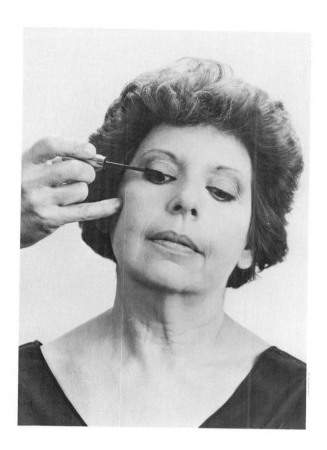

Photo 8
Mascara is brushed on to thicken and beautify the lashes. It is first applied to the lower lashes. The eyes should be opened, looking upward for ease of application. The client looks down when the mascara is brushed onto the upper lashes. Two applications may be needed to achieve the desired result.

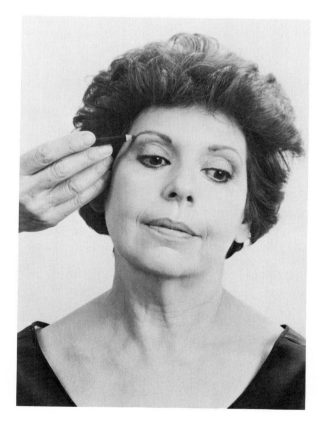

Photo 9
Brow pencil is used to give shape to the brows. Sketch on little hair-like strokes with the pencil. Use a very sharp pointed lead to achieve a natural look. If the pencil strokes are obvious apply a touch of powder to the brows and then fluff off excess.

Photo 10

A soft accent blush is now applied. Use a shade in the same color category as the lipstick. Soft rose, pink and mocha are good choices. The blush is first applied under the cheek bone and then brought up onto the fullness of the cheeks. If a cream blush is used it should have been applied before the powder.

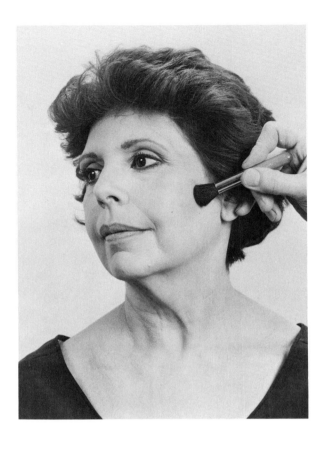

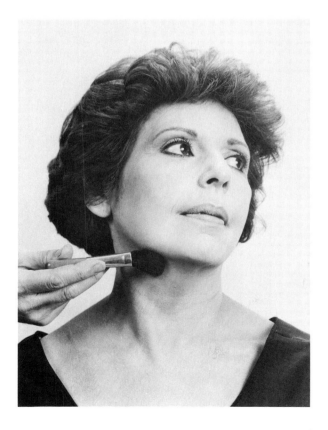

Photo 11

To strengthen the jawline and diminish fullness under the chin, a tawny or fawn blush is applied directly under the jawline and runs from a point under one ear to the other.

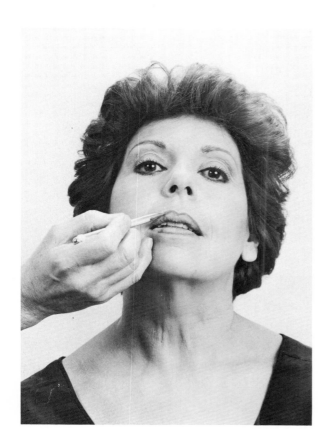

Photo 12

To outline the lips, use a color in the same category as the lipstick but a shade or two deeper. To steady your hand, rest your small finger on the model's chin. Starting from the lip corner away from you, draw the line following the natural lip contour on the upper and lower lips.

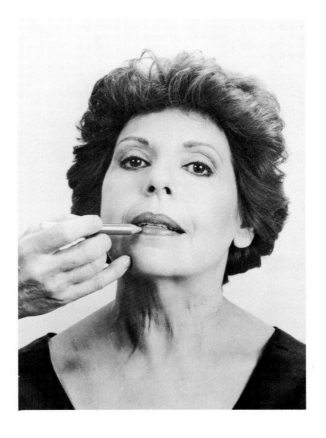

Photo 13

With the lips drawn in a semi-smile and slightly parted, fill in with the lip color, blending it onto the lip line that has been drawn in.

If the model has little lines around the lips that may cause a bleeding of the lipstick, you might use the lip pencil to color the entire lip area. As it is made of a harder wax than lipstick it will not bleed past the lip outline. A colorless lip gloss may be applied to the center of the lips to add sheen.

Cosmetic face-lift

Photo 14
Face tapes are being applied to the areas in front of the ears and at the temples.

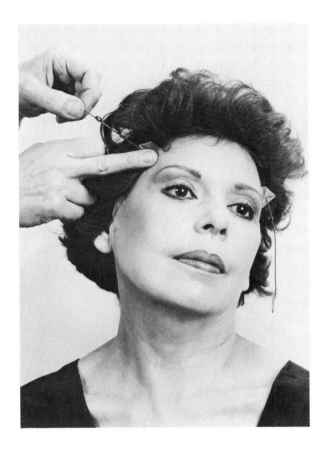

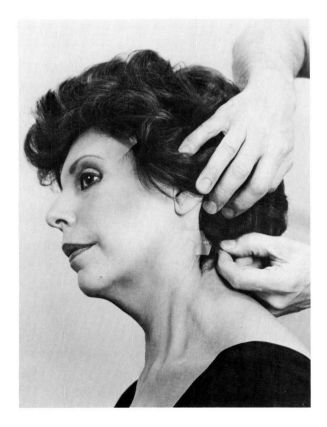

Photo 15
Tapes for the neck are being applied. This will smooth out the neck line area. (See chapter 6—Face Lifting Techniques.)

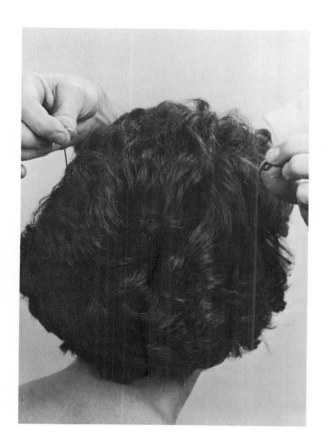

Photo 16
The elastics from the tapes are being drawn to the top of the crown of the head and fastened. Neck tapes are very short and are hidden by the hair at the nape line.

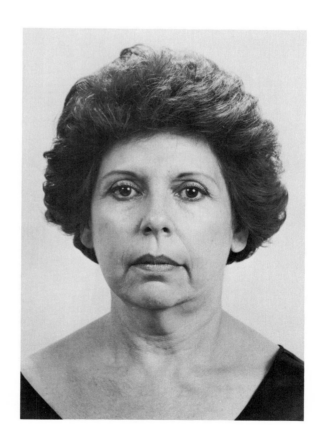

Photo 17
By looking at this "before" photo and at the following "after" photo you can plainly see that make-up and our little beauty secret (lifts) can help the mature woman maintain a youthful look.

Photo 18
We see our model here looking fresh and flawless. Of course not everyone would want face tapes applied, but for professional models and actresses it is a perfect solution to eliminating wrinkles temporarily.

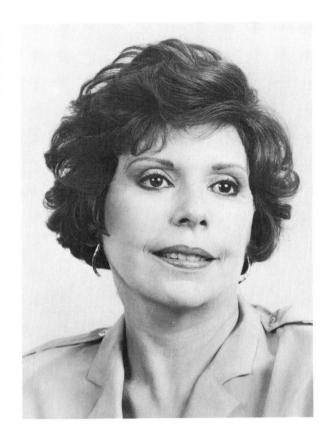

Chapter 12

Creating a
Look of Fashion

The term "High Fashion" paints in the minds of most people the picture of an ultra sophisticated woman. She is standing in a somewhat dramatic pose, wearing designer clothes and made-up in an equally dramatic manner. Though this may sometimes be true, "high fashion" in reality alludes to that which is considered the epitome of the very newest fashion at the time. Sometimes the "in" look may be very natural and casual, and must too be considered "high fashion."

Fashion of course changes with the seasons and what is considered chic this year may be very dated in another six months. To create a look of fashion we chose to go back in time for inspiration to the very exciting era of the 1920's. Picture the flapper with her short skirts, cupid's bow lip, and shingled bob hairdo. Understand, we did not wish to do an exact duplicate of the look but rather modify and update it. As a matter of fact, many famous designers use their textbook knowledge of the history of costume, hairstyling and make-up to help them create their contemporary works of beauty.

For this venture into restyling, we chose as our model the renowned fashion make-up artist Sherne, who is as well known for her frequent radical change of looks as she is for her make-up expertise. On the pages that follow, you will see how one individual can affect many different looks, all through the simple application of make-up.

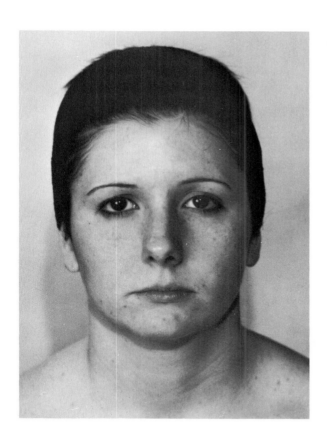

APPLICATION OF MAKE-UP

Photo 1

Although Sherne's features have a very distinctive look, her well spaced eyes, thin brows and small features lend themselves to a variety of changes.

Photo 2

A porcelain toned underbase is applied before the application of a creamy ivory fluid make-up base. The look we seek is a pale almost translucent skin tone. Both the toner and the base are applied to the face, lids, lips and then down onto the neck area.

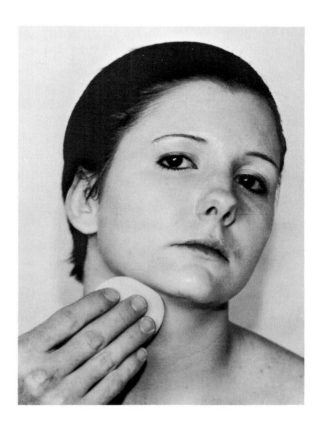

Photo 3

A pale translucent powder, brushed on evenly, gives a matte smooth finish to the complexion.

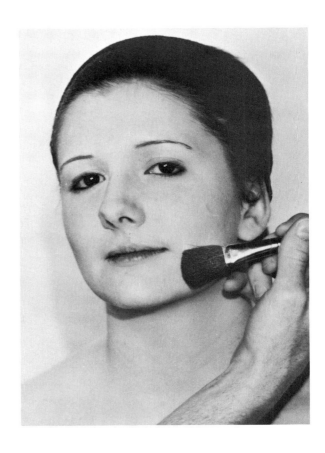

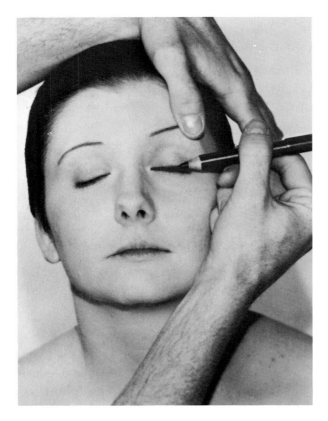

Photo 4

Black liner crayon is applied down at the base of the lashes. One hand holds the lid taut while the liner is drawn from near the inner corner out to the outer corner of the eye.

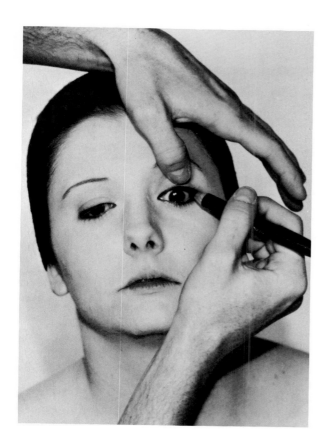

Photo 5

The model is told to look downward while the eyelid is held open. This holds the eye muscle steady while liner is applied to the inner platform of the eye (directly at the under base of the upper lashes).

This extends from the inner to outer eye corner. Do this carefully and quickly so as to disturb the client as little as possible.

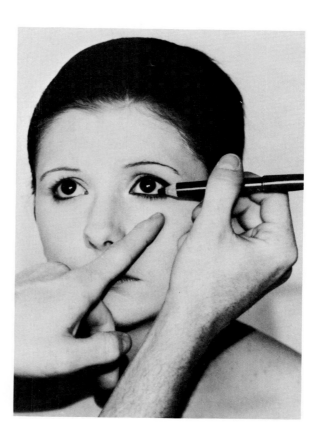

Photo 6

The black liner is then applied to the lower lid area. It is first applied to the inner platform of the lid (directly above the lower lashes), again running the line from the inner to outer corner. Liner is then placed below this line directly to the base of the lower lashes. This lower line should be softened somewhat by running a sponge shadow applicator or cotton swab across in a smudging effect.

Photo 7

The eyelid is designed in three steps:

1. Black eye-shadow is brushed on the crease or depth area. It starts one fourth of the distance out from the inner corner to past the outer corner where it is applied more heavily.
2. The eyelid itself is shadowed with a magenta tint.
3. The center of the lid has a pink highlighting shadow. The black shadow meets the liner at the outer corner forming a horizontal 'V' shape.

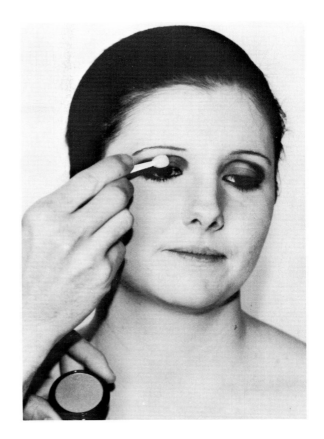

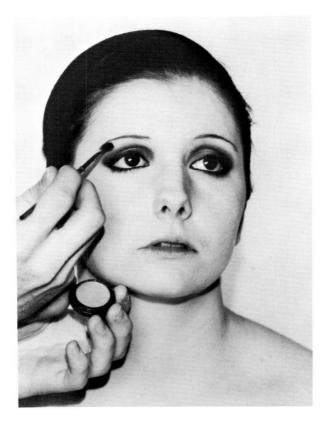

Photo 8

A pale shimmer of lavender eye-shadow highlights the brow bone.

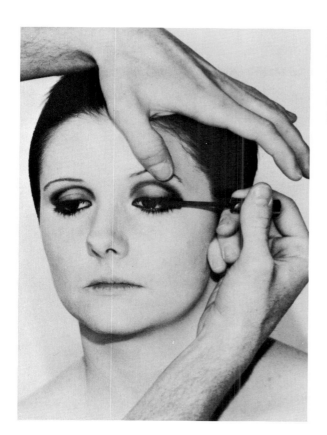

Photo 9
Black mascara is applied to both the lower and upper lashes. Three applications of mascara to the top lashes add a dramatic look. After each application the lashes are separated with a lash brush to keep them from caking together.

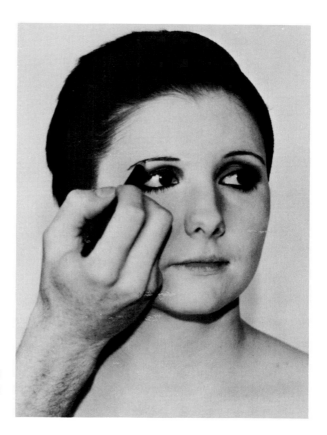

Photo 10
The thin eyebrows are simply sketched with a dark brown pencil to accentuate but not thicken their delicate look.

Photo 11
Magenta blush is merely hinted at in the hollow of the cheek. With the eyes and lips to be the focus of attention, it is wise to play down the cheek area.

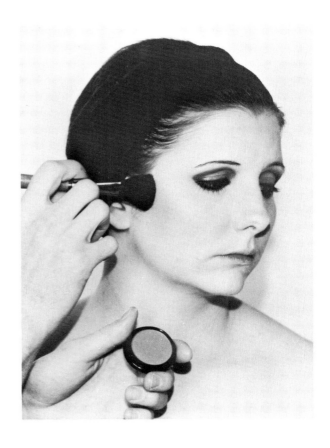

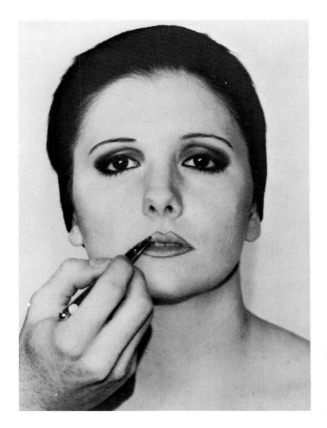

Photo 12
A deep red lip liner pencil is used to outline the lips. Our model's naturally thin lips are slightly extended particularly to emphasize the lip bow.

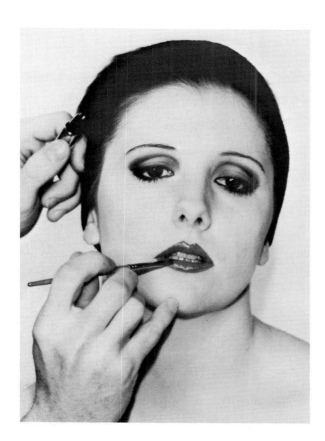

Photo 13
Lipstick in a coordinated wine-red shade is brushed on to give the lips a smooth and shiny look.

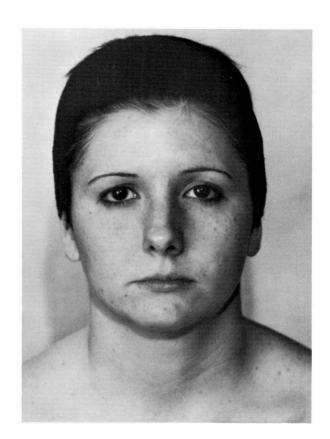

Photo 14
Returning to our "before" photo and then glancing at the following finished "looks" points up the enormous difference that a change of make-up and hairstyles can make.

116

Photo 15
Coiffure in place, the 'total look' is completed. A dramatic statement of fashion of yesterday, today or tomorrow.

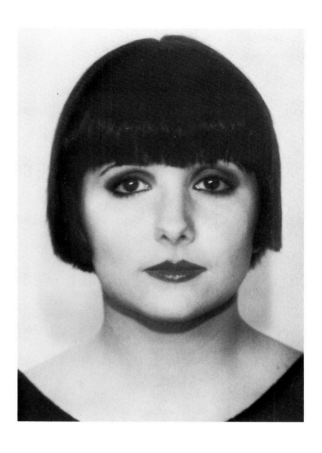

Here is Sherne in some of her other moods. A change of hair color, hair style and a change of make-up, helps create many different moods, from sweet to soignee. It's just a matter of beauty expertise.

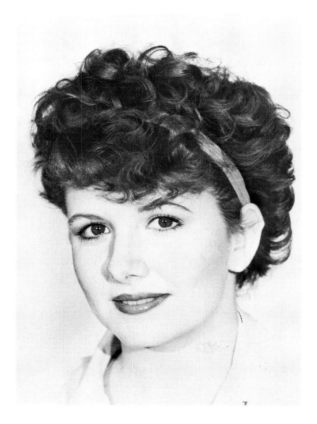

Photo 16
Sweet Simplicity

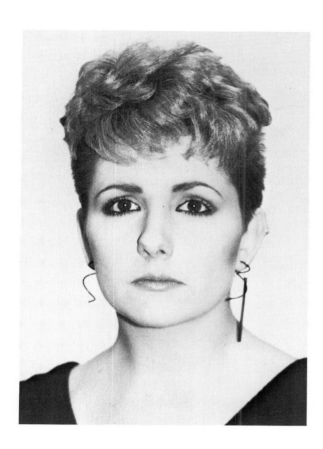

Photo 17
Executive Suite

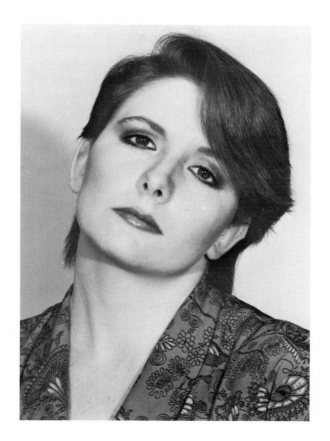

Photo 18
Ever Romantic

Photo 19
Look of the 80's

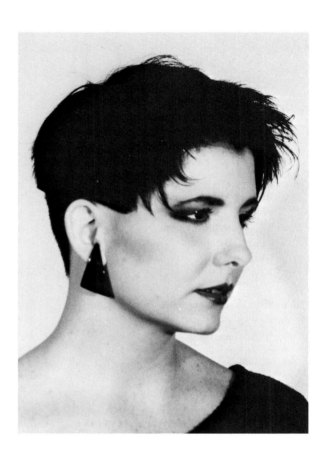

Chapter 13

Make-up for Men

SPECIAL CONSIDERATIONS

Make-up for men, no matter for what occasion or media, should always have one aim. The make-up must look as natural as possible and in fact should look as if no make-up was used. Many male models use no make-up at all when being photographed for fashion magazines. If the skin is very pale they may choose to use a suntan base. Shadows under the eyes may be eliminated with a cover-up and pale brows might be darkened slightly, but in general very little make-up is used. For television and film more make-up is used but again it must be applied carefully and must look very natural. In the following photos the model was made-up for stage and for intimate or mid-range theatre.

SPECIAL HINTS

- For larger theatres, the make-up can be somewhat stronger by contouring the eyes and highlighting and shading the features for better delineation.

- For film and television, the make-up must be more subdued and liner and mascara should look nonexistant even on close scrutiny.

- For television, do not use lip color.

The following pages illustrate the special techniques that are unique to making-up men for the stage or film.

APPLICATION OF MAKE-UP

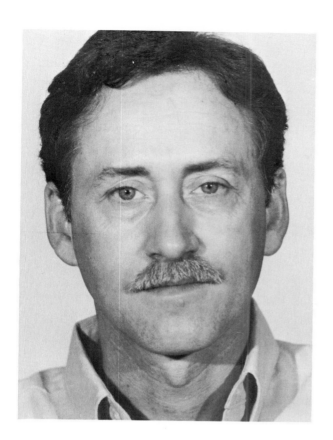

Photo 1
Our model has fairly good coloring but in stage lighting he would look very washed out without make-up. His mustache is quite blonde in contrast to his brown hair and his brows and lashes can stand darkening.

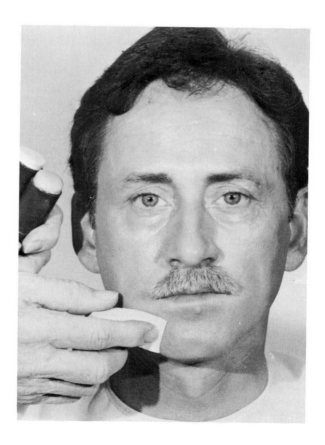

Photo 2
Two shades of cream stick are used to create just the coloring desired. This is only done when the exact shade is not available. Both sticks are held together in one hand and the sponge wisks across them picking up a bit of color from both. The make-up is applied in a thin application over the entire face, eyelids, ears and down to the neck.

Photo 3

A base about three shades lighter is applied in the shadows under the eye puffs. This might also be done more carefully using a light cover-up and applied with a small brush. Any shadows or blemishes can be neutralized this way.

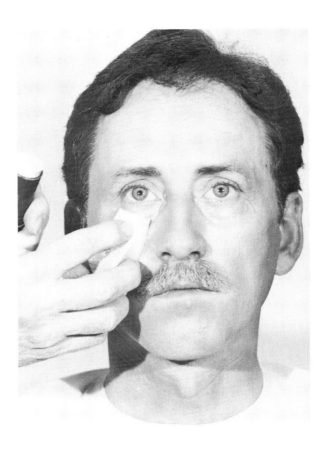

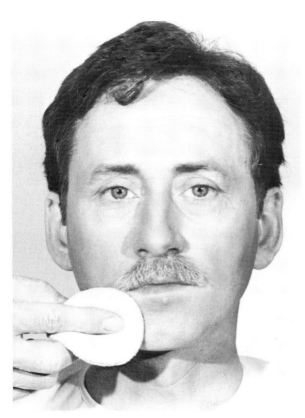

Photo 4

With the skin tone evened out, the face is powdered with a translucent powder. Using a large velour puff, dip into the powder container and rub the powder into the puff by folding it together. Rub so the powder permeates the puff. Then press the powder onto the face to set the make-up.

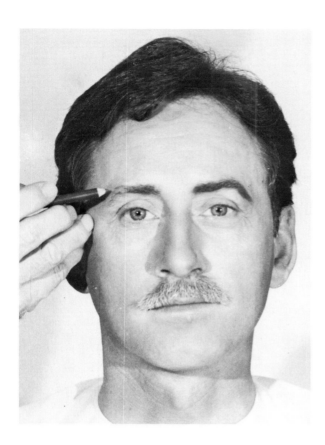

Photo 5
Eyebrows are filled in with a brown shade of pencil to match the hair color.

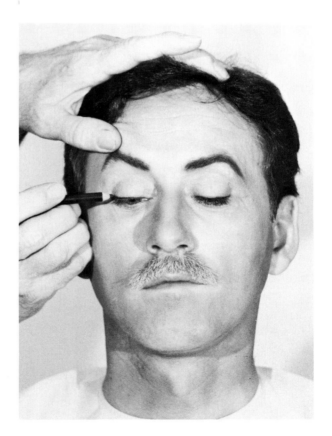

Photo 6
Brown eye-liner pencil is used to create a line directly in and above the top lashes.

Photo 7
Use a shadow applicator or cotton swab to smudge the line blending it down into the lash base.

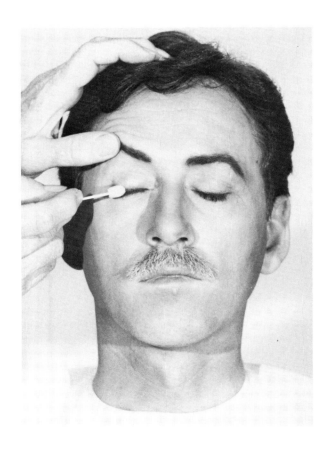

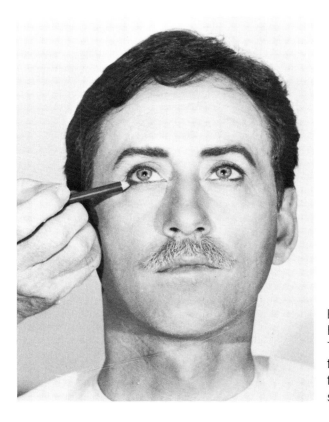

Photo 8
Eye-liner is applied to the bottom lashes also. The pencil is run from the outer corner in toward the inner corner gradually diminishing about three quarters of the way in. This line is also smudged to soften it.

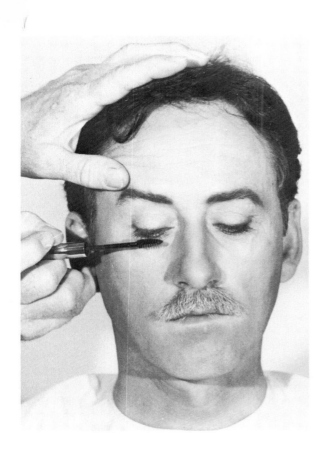

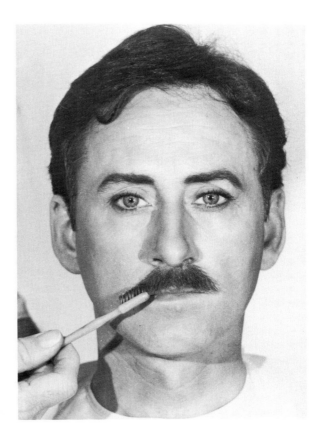

Photo 9
Brown mascara is used to emphasize the top and lower lashes. Just one application and then the lashes are brushed through with a clean lash brush to separate the lashes and make sure the mascara is not obvious.

Photo 10
A brown pencil is rubbed across a small brush and then applied to the mustache to darken it to the hair color.

Photo 11
A slight cleft in the chin is deepened with brown pencil to add interest to the face.

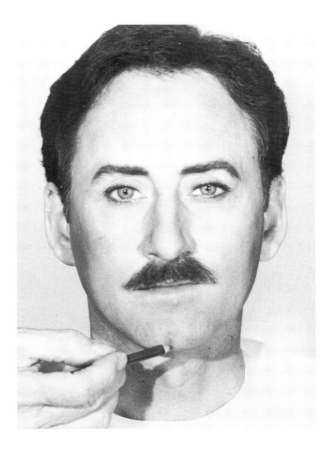

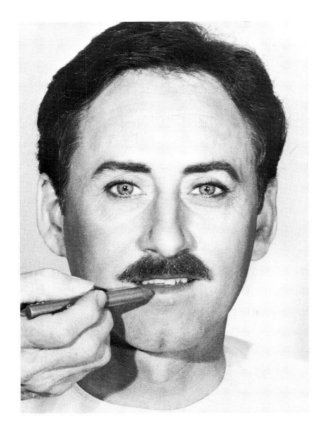

Photo 12
For the stage, a lip color is added to the lips to deepen them so they do not wash out in the stage lighting. The color should be a very natural tawny shade.

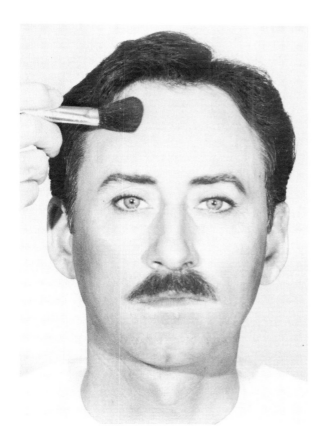

Photo 13
A tawny shade of blush with a rose cast or a bronze shade is brushed across the forehead, cheeks, chin, and nose to give color dimension to the face. This is done if deemed necessary.

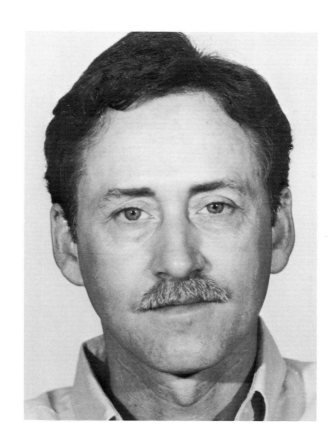

Photo 14
Is there any doubt after looking at this "before" photo and then at the following "after" photo that men can benefit from a judicial application of make-up?

Photo 15
Here is the finished make-up. Contrast this with the first photo and see how the face comes alive and how the features are so much more outstanding with make-up than without.

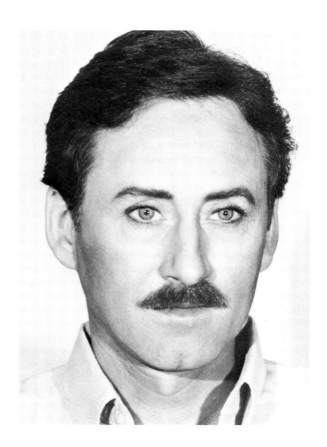

Chapter 14

Aging the Face
With Make-up

It is often necessary for a model, actor or actress to look older or appear more mature than they are. To make someone look only slightly older it is only necessary to add a few lines or shadows to suggest the difference in age. This is usually sufficient for most media. When it is necessary to make someone look twenty to thirty years older, however, more effort must be taken. Highlighting and shading may be enough for stage or some photography but for film which is much more demanding, prosthetics are usually used. These are foamed latex features that are made expressly for the actor or actress and look realistic even to the searching eye of the close-up camera.

SPECIAL CONSIDERATIONS

The younger the subject, the more difficult it is to do a realistic aging with highlighting and shading. However, for the somewhat mature face it is not a difficult procedure. Using the same model we used for the chapter on make-up for men, we proceeded to do an aging make-up. On the following pages you will see the gradual aging process with simple make-up application.

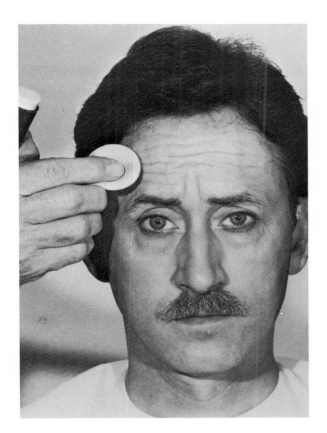

APPLICATION OF MAKE-UP

Photo 1
An appropriate cream make-up was first applied to the face. Every line and wrinkle in the face has a shadow and a highlight. The depth of the wrinkle is dark and the surrounding area is light. Have the model make faces by wrinkling the various areas of the face. Here the forehead is lifted to form lines and a foundation about three shades lighter than the base is drawn downward in a sweeping movement leaving horizontal forehead lines. Do the same for the other facial areas such as frown lines and crow's feet around the eyes.

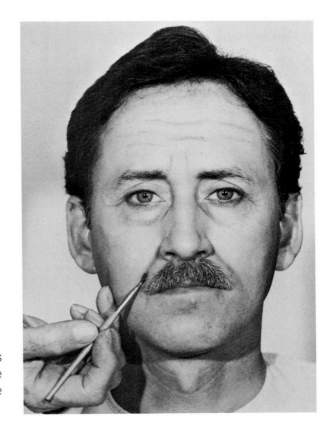

Photo 2
Using a base four or five shades deeper, lines are deepened with a small flat brush. Here the naso-labial fold is emphasized by darkening the depth area.

Photo 3
The same thing is done to create stronger lines on the forehead, under-the-eye puffs, the frown lines, the eye fold and the inner corner or the eye area. The lines should be softened and blended.

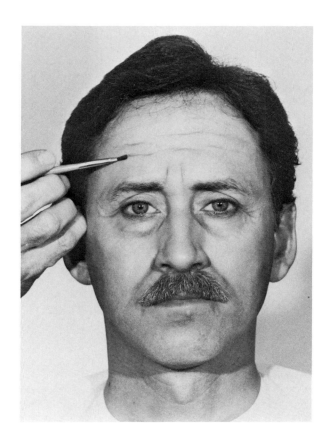

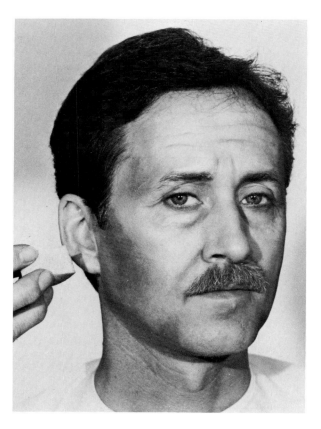

Photo 4
Using a sponge and the shading base we deepen the temporal area, hollow the cheeks and create the look of jowls by darkening the sides of the chin.

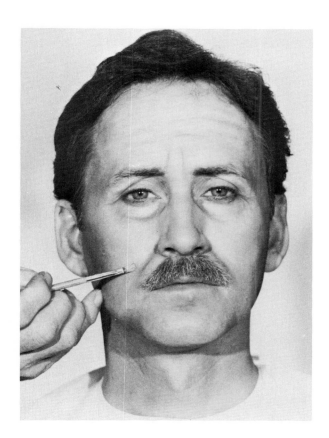

Photo 5
Switching back to the highlighting base, we paint directly above the darkened naso-labial fold. The fold of the brow bone is also highlighted to suggest a falling eyelid.

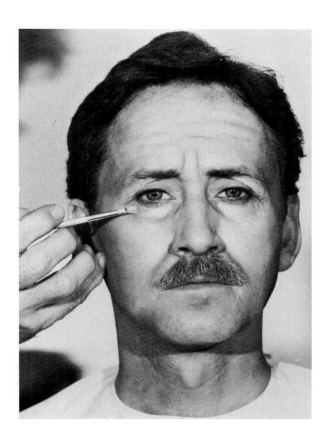

Photo 6
The eye puffs are highlighted as is the area between the vertical frown lines.

Photo 7
Small lines are drawn on and around the lips with a brown pencil. Lines are also drawn around the outer corner of the lips and on the bottom of the chin. In the finished make-up this will give the chin and lips a lined and mottled appearance.

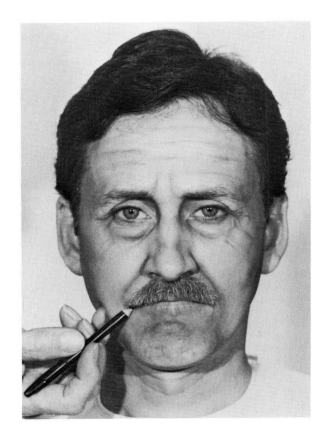

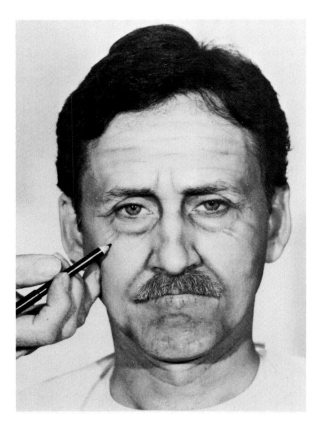

Photo 8
The lines surrounding the eyes are also deepened, as are any other lines that require it.

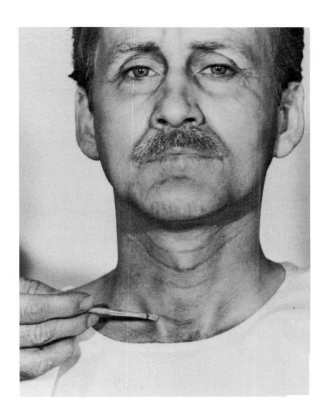

Photo 9
Do not neglect the neck area. Deep lines have been sketched in and the highlight is now being applied.

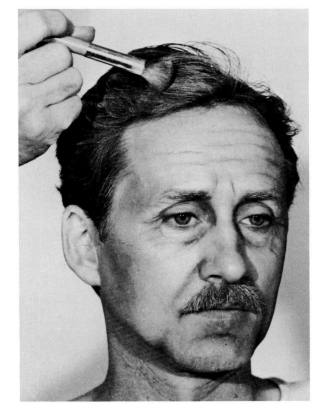

Photo 10
The face has been powdered down with a regular translucent powder. Pictured here, white powder is being brushed through the hair for a grey appearance. For a hair whitening which will last through an evening stage appearance it would be necessary to use a regular hair whitener in cream or liquid form.

Photo 11
This "before" photo, with corrective make-up applied, and then the following finished "aging make-up" certainly emphasizes the importance of make-up for the stage.

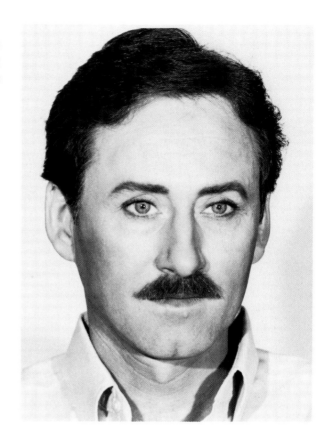

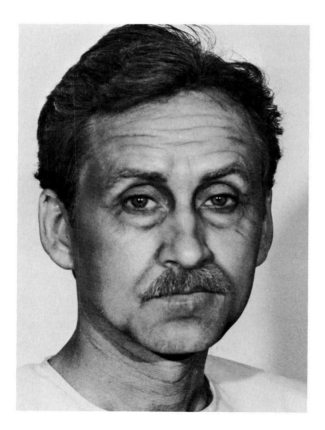

Photo 12
With a quizzical look on his face, our model stares at himself in the mirror.

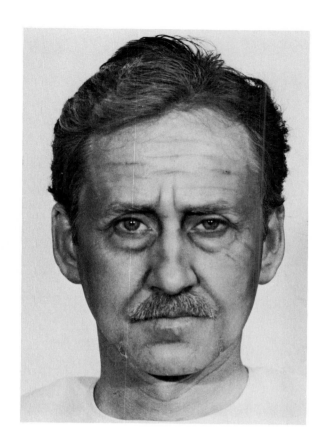

Photo 13
In another view, notice how the make-up helps the actor project various emotions. Of course if the part to be played is not quite this old then the make-up should be applied lighter and fewer lines emphasized.

Chapter 15

How to Create a Beard and Mustache

There are several ways in which beards may be attached to the face. If the beard is for the stage and is to be worn night after night or if it is to be worn in a film, the best type is one made of real hair that is ventilated (individually knotted) onto a lace foundation. These are easy to apply and look very realistic but they do take some time to make and are fairly expensive.

PRODUCTS USED FOR MAKING BEARDS AND MUSTACHES

For use in a one time application for amateur theatricals, a print ad or television appearance, where the camera does not come in too close, a beard made of crepe wool is popularly used. Crepe wool, sometimes called crepe hair, is quite economical, and fairly easy to apply with practice. This type of beard must be applied to the face each time it is needed and can only be used once, unless it is applied to a latex base. The standard method is to use spirit gum, just as when applying the ventilated beard type. Crepe wool is also used for sideburns, eyebrows, mustaches and even to fill in receding hairlines.

This product comes in braids of kinky wool strands tied together with string. It comes in various shades such as white, black, red, blond, and several shades of gray and brown. For the most realistic effect, several shades of compatible colors should be used. For example, in a black beard you might achieve a more natural effect if you blend in either red or brown with some gray if need be. In a blond beard you might mix in some light brown, red, or even white. Mixing is done after having straightened the hair. The pages that follow explain the techniques for preparing the materials used for artificial facial hair and how they are applied.

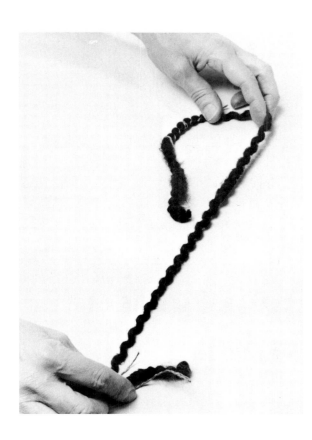

APPLICATION OF A BEARD

Photo 1

To prepare the crepe wool, first undo the braid by cutting the string that holds it together. Dampen the portion of hair to be used. If there is time, stretch the hair between two solid forms such as the arms or legs of a chair and leave it to dry overnight. Since not all facial hair is straight (a curly haired man is bound to have at least some curl or wave to his beard), only straighten the hair to the degree desired.

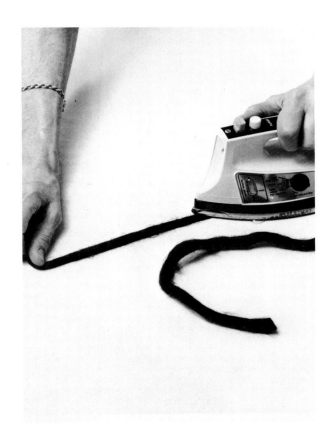

Photo 2

A fast way to straighten the crepe hair is with a steam iron. If you are not using a steam iron, make sure to place a damp cloth over the hair to prevent scorching.

Photo 3

Knowing we were going to create a very short beard, we cut the sections to about four inches long. For beginners, a longer length is easier to handle. Much depends on the finished length of beard you wish to create. The pieces are now being spread out in thinned layers. It is a good idea to make a sketch of the shape and size of the desired beard and mustache before starting so that you will know how much hair you may need and what length to cut the sections.

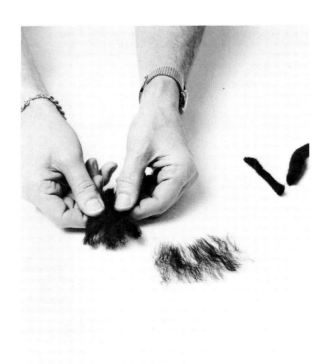

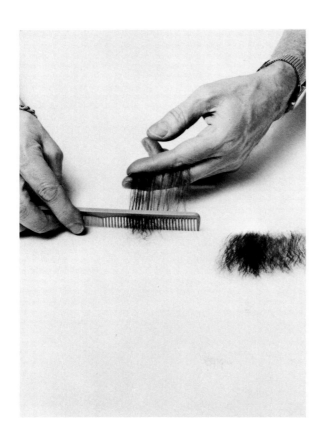

Photo 4

For our model we are using both medium brown and dark brown hair. The two shades are blended, combed together and laid out in neat rows ready for use.

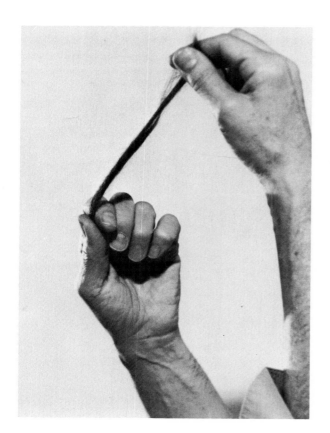

Photo 5
Another and perhaps more simple way to prepare hair for a beard is to start out with strands from 5 to 7 inches in length. This method is particularly good when preparing for a longer type beard. First hold one strand at one end and gently tug strands loose from the other end. Lay this layer down and then use the same technique to remove strands from the second shade. Lay this down over the first group. In this way you will be mixing your colors.

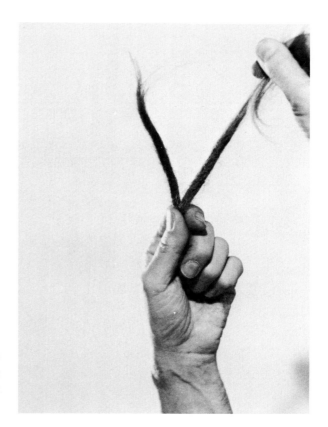

Photo 6
You may also try holding both shades at the same time and pulling some hairs from one strand and some from the other making an automatic mix of the colors.

Photo 7
Here are the longer strands, premixed and ready to be applied.

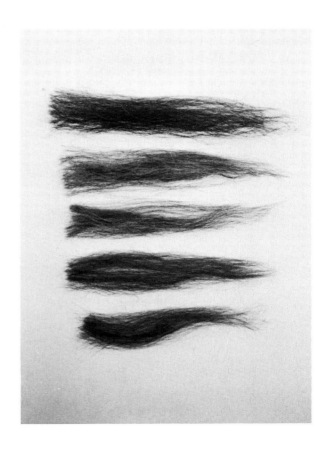

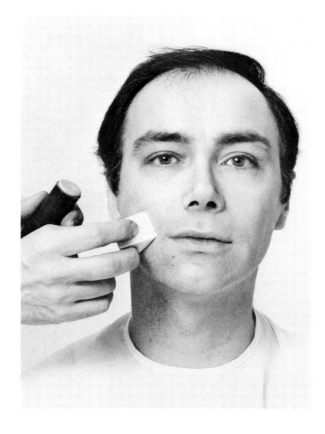

Photo 8
The basic make-up is applied. A cake type make-up is often best to use since prosthetics and beards do not cling well to a greasy surface. Since our model prefers a cream stick type of base, we apply only a very thin layer of make-up.

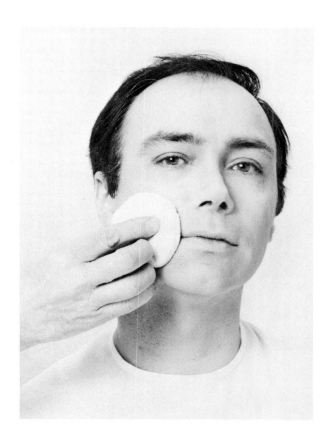

Photo 9
Since we used a cream make-up, it is required that the skin be powdered down very well to supply a dry surface for the beard application.

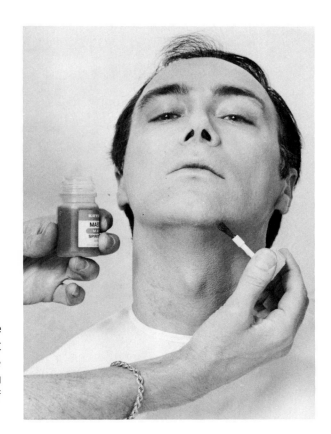

Photo 10
The usual start of the application is the underside of the chin. An application of spirit gum is applied to an area of perhaps 2 to 2½ inches in width and ½ inch in thickness. As you begin to work, you will determine the amount of hair you can handle comfortably.

Photo 11

Separate a small portion of hair, not too thick, and trim the edge that is to be attached to the skin. All trimming of the hair that is to go against the face must be trimmed in advance of placement as it cannot be done once it is glued to the skin.

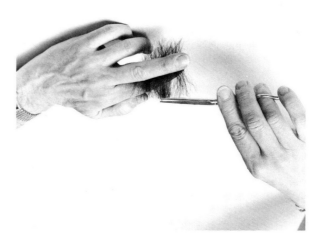

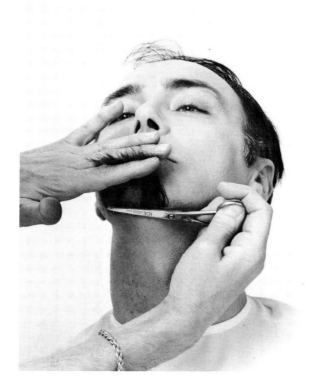

Photo 12

The hair is placed against the underside of the chin and pressed on firmly with the scissors. As you work, make sure you keep the scissors clean by cleaning them occasionally with acetone and wiping them dry.

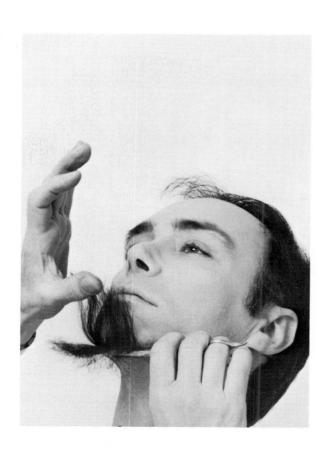

Photo 13
Working back from the point of the chin, apply perhaps two or three more sections, each time applying the spirit gum first and then laying on the hair. Spirit gum does not dry completely so it is not necessary to work fast. Take your time to do a perfect job.

Photo 14
After the underside of the chin is finished, begin at the front of the chin and work upwards, again in layers. Trim the hair to be placed against the skin to the desired shape.

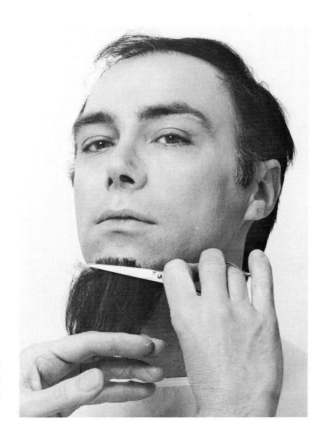

146

Photo 15

If you are applying a full beard, the next area to be covered is the underside of the jaw. Always follow the natural hair growth which is more or less vertical with a slight angle at the jaw area. Start at a point under the jawline and work in pieces upward and forward until you blend the hair into the hair on the chin. In this photo the section is cut to fit in with the top shaping of the beard and glued on in a vertical manner angled ever so slightly forward.

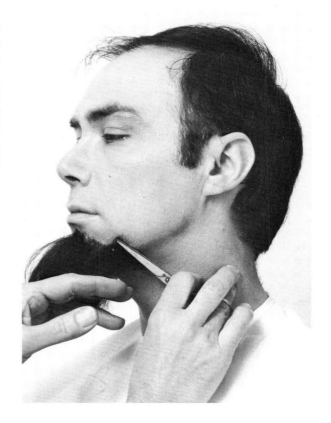

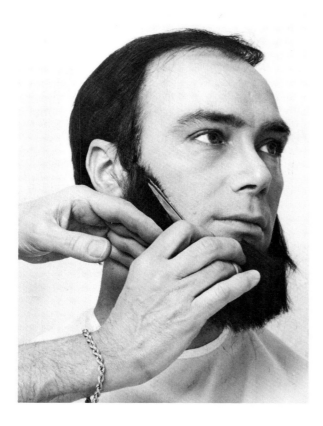

Photo 16

Section after section has been applied, first under the jaw and then layered on top until the sideburn is reached.

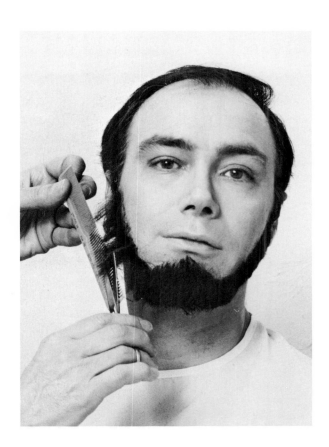

Photo 17
Before applying the mustache, we decided to do our basic cutting of the beard to see how it looked. Extreme caution must be used to avoid cutting it too short. Trim it little by little until you have just the correct style.

Photo 18
Mustaches can be applied in one, two or even four sections to each side. It depends on your dexterity and the type of mustache desired. We placed one layer close to the lip first. The photo shows the second layer being applied above the first.

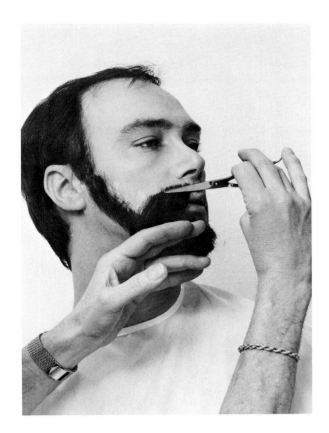

Photo 19
Pressing the beard with a lint free cloth may be done several times during the creation of the facial hair. It helps hair adhere to the face.

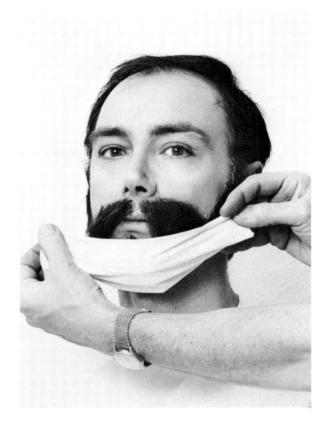

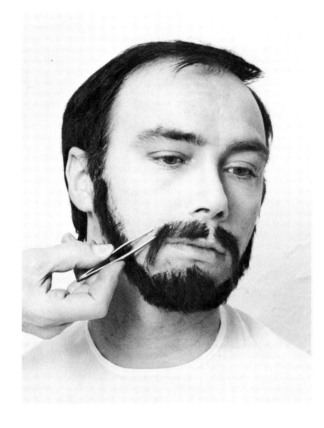

Photo 20
After the final trimming of the beard and mustache, (make sure you place a finger against the lip when trimming the mustache to avoid cutting the lip) the hair may be combed very lightly with a wide-toothed comb to remove loose hairs. You can then fill in with bits of hair along the hairline where needed, or as seen in this photo, vagrant hairs may be removed with a tweezer. The edge of the beard should not look too solid in order to avoid a very heavy or artificial look.

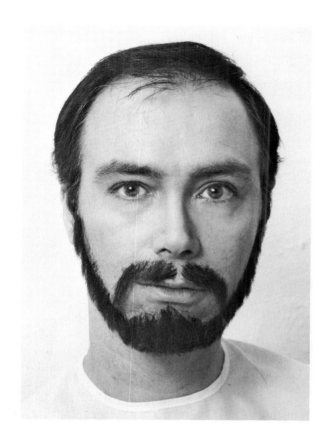

Photo 21

The finished facial hair looks fairly natural even in this close-up. If the spirit gum appears too shiny then try using a matte finish adhesive which has less of a shine. Though it is not quite as strong as the regular spirit gum it does the job well enough.

You may spray longer beards lightly with hair spray and form the beard and mustache with your hands to give it better shape. Be sure to cover the eyes and nose when using spray on the beard.

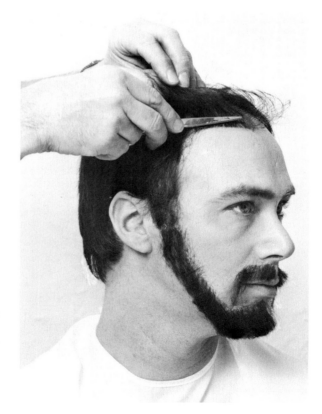

Photo 22

Crepe hair may be used for other purposes such as eyebrows, sideburns and even filling in hairlines. In this photo you can see a layer of crepe hair being placed at the forehead hairline. Of course we filled in the back area first and then worked forward.

Photo 23
Let's take a glimpse of our model before we started.

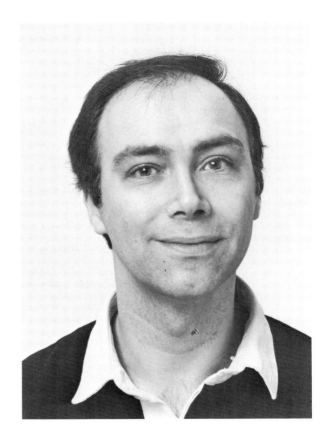

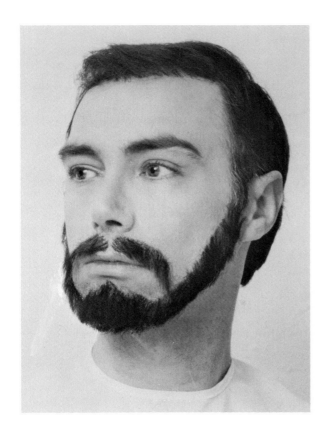

Photo 24
Here he is with a neat, trimmed beard and a corrected hairline. Indeed a very dapper and handsome appearance.

Crepe hair can also be used for beard stubble to give an unshaven look. In this type of application the face is washed with soap and water and then cleansed of all grease with an astringent. The crepe hair is cut up into tiny pieces on a sheet of paper. Apply mustache wax or stubble paste to the beard area, the mustache area and under the jawline down onto the neck. Attach the bits of crepe hair to the face with a powder brush by dipping it into the cut up pieces and spreading it evenly on the skin. Beard stubble can be removed with cleansing cream or make-up remover.

Eyebrows can be augmented or entirely new brows constructed with crepe hair. To make the brows heavier or to change their shape, attach the crepe hair to the skin above the brow with spirit gum and comb it down into the brow.

Chapter 16

Special Effects With Three-Dimensional Products

Although it is possible to suggest changes in features through the use of cosmetics by highlighting, shading and coloring, it is not a satisfactory way to literally change, say, the nose, chin or cheeks. To change a feature and also to create the three-dimensional effect of raised bruises, scars or deeply lined skin, it is necessary to use special make-up products. These cosmetics are available wherever theatrical make-up is sold.

PRODUCTS USED FOR SPECIAL EFFECTS

1. **Spirit Gum** is used as an adhesive for attaching various products to the skin. It comes in liquid form and is available in both regular and matte finish.

2. **Derma Wax** is useful for building features such as the nose, chin, and raised bruises. It is also used to create scars and skin irregularities and also to cover eyebrows.

3. **Plastic Sealer** is used to firm and coat wax features. Flexible collodion may also be used.

4. **Scarring Material** is primarily used to simulate old scars or cuts in the skin. Non-flexible collodion may also be used for this purpose.

5. **Liquid Latex** helps create a natural looking aged skin. It is also useful for creating small latex pieces (prosthetics).

6. **Stipple Sponge** is a small, square wiry type sponge that gives texture to wax features.

Changing the features of the actress or actor to suit the character they are portraying can be lots of fun to do. Using the above products will give you satisfactory results but remember that it must be repeated for each performance. When the facial change is called for night after night or if the make-up is being created for film, much more elaborate and technically perfect make-up is required. The skills required to create realistic looking prosthetics made usually from foamed latex take much study and experience to aquire. Let us first become proficient at simpler and more accessible methods of character make-up.

CHANGING THE SHAPE OF THE NOSE

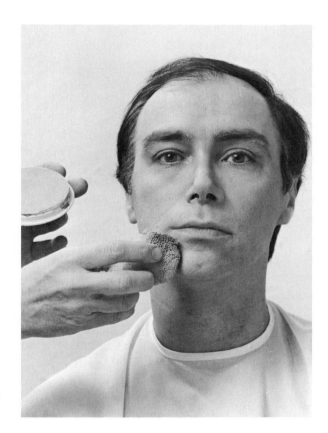

Photo 1
We persuaded our model to let us use cake make-up rather than his favorite cream base. We chose a color very close to his own and applied it with a dampened natural sponge. It is not necessary to powder down cake make-up.

Photo 2

After deciding what type of nose we will be creating, we painted a layer of spirit gum within the area the wax will be placed. If you wish, you might even outline this area with a brow pencil.

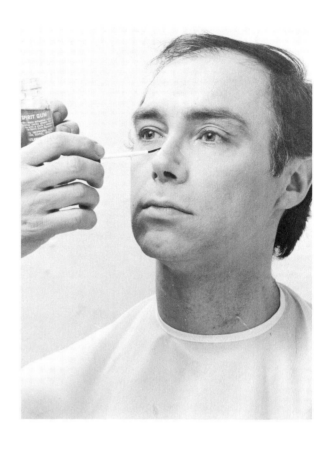

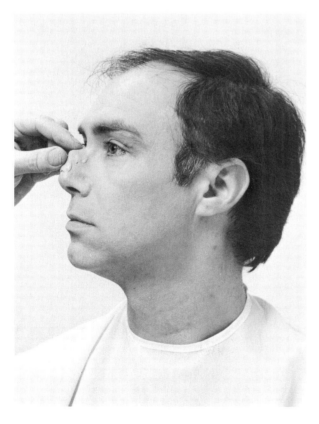

Photo 3

A small amount of wax has been placed within this outline and is being spread and shaped. If you find that the wax is sticking to your fingers, dip your fingers into hair styling gel. This will keep the wax from clinging to them.

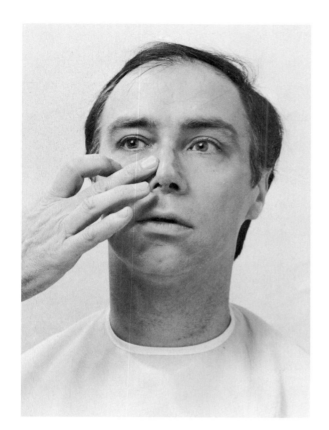

Photo 4
The fingertips are used to sculpture and model the feature. Keep in mind not to use too much wax (at least not more than is called for) and do not spread the wax past the designing outline.

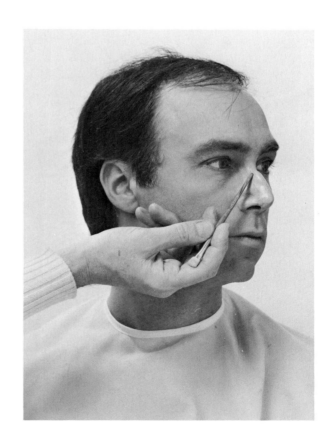

Photo 5
Any kind of modeling tool may be used that will be helpful in creating the desired effect. Here we are using the handle end of a brush. A plastic spatula can be a big help also.

Photo 6

Brush on one or two layers of sealer on the wax once you have the finished nose shape. If the person has generally fine skin, the pore effect should be very slight. To indicate a rough textured skin, perhaps on a mature or a sun-weathered skin, a deeply pored texture may be called for. Use a stipple sponge for this purpose.

A cream base in the same shade as the tone used on the skin should be gently pressed on the wax nose. If needed, a shade deeper may be used. The nose should then be powdered down.

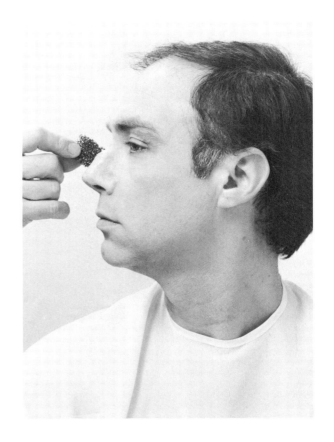

CREATING A RAISED BRUISE WITH OPEN CUT

Photo 7

Spirit gum is again applied to the area where we desire the bruise.

In this photo the wax has been placed within this area, pressed down firmly into the spirit gum, and spread with the finger tips. The edges have been blended carefully. Remember that if the wax sticks to the fingers, the use of a little hairstyling gel will solve the problem. Sometimes just dampening the fingers with water will help or even the use of a tiny bit of moisturizing cream will suffice. Keep wiping the fingers clean as you work.

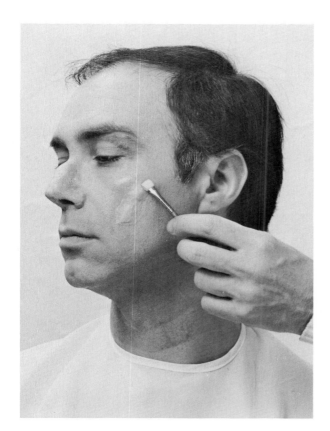

Photo 8
This time we are smoothing and blending the edges with the help of a sponge-tipped shadow applicator. You see, almost any tool at hand can be of help.

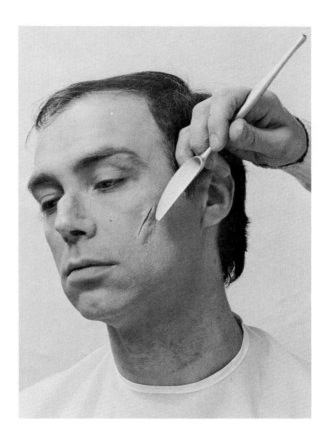

Photo 9
An old, very dull butter knife or a spatula will help open the wax if an open cut is the desired effect. Apply a coat of the sealer and allow it to dry. Next, color the wax with the same color base as used on the skin.

Photo 10
If you wish to make it appear as a fresh cut, paint on some stage blood or even red cream rouge.

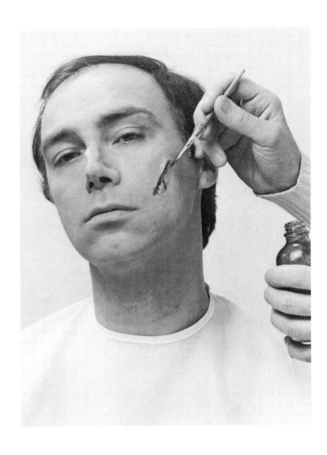

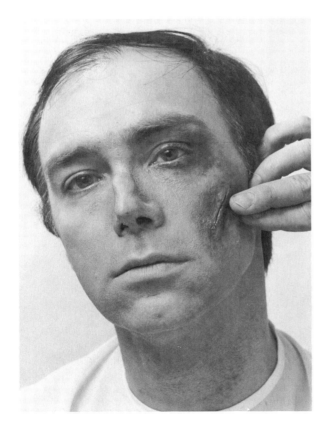

Photo 11
For the look of a bad bruise with a slightly healed cut, the blood is omitted and the wax is discolored with purple and maroon shading to add a look of authenticity. The eye is slightly discolored also.

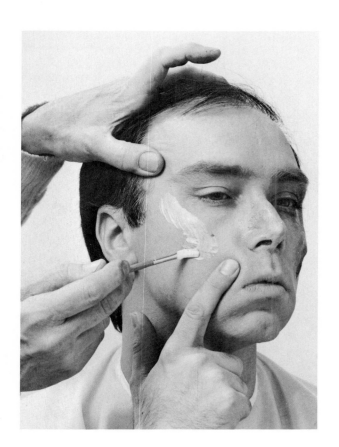

CREATING DEEPLY BURNT OR DEFORMED SKIN

For this effect we will use liquid latex, tissue, powder and a hair dryer.

Photo 12
Before applying the latex you may use some moisturizer or even a little baby oil on the skin. This is to protect the skin if it is sensitive. Blot off all the excess before proceeding and powder the area. Here we see the latex being applied to the area we want to wrinkle. The skin must be held taut during the entire process. The model holds the skin pulling downward and the artist stretches the skin upward. Drawing the skin vertically will cause the skin to wrinkle and fold horizontally. The opposite is true when you wish to create vertical wrinkles. The skin then must be stretched horizontally.

Photo 13
Tear a single layer of tissue to fit exactly over the area where the latex was painted. Do not cut the tissue but rather allow it to have rough edges. Again paint latex directly over the tissue, first painting over the edges and then over the entire area. Do not allow the latex to touch the hair either on the brows or hairline as it would be difficult to remove. Remember that the skin must be held taut the entire time.

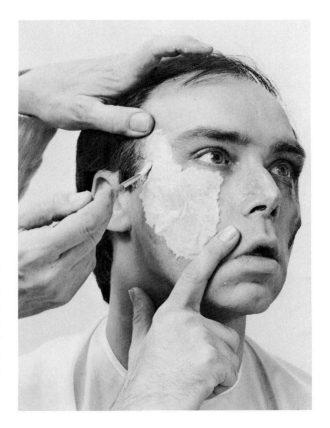

Photo 14

The latex is now dried with a blow dryer. The heat should not be too warm as it will dry fast enough. Still holding the skin taut, powder is brushed over the area when the latex is dry. The skin can be allowed to relax to form folds. Make-up is now pressed over the latexed area in a color which matches the general skin tone.

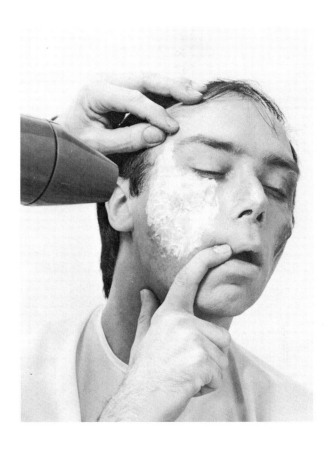

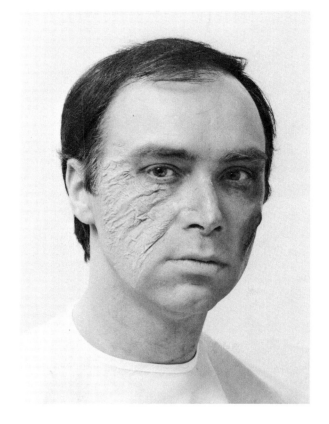

Photo 15

Here we see the effects of the disfigured skin. Listed below are the different looks you can create using this technique with a few modifications.

A. For the look of skin badly damaged by a fire or radioactive burn, the area should be colored with tints of red, purple and maroon. This will give a raw damaged appearance.

B. For a freshly burned effect, pull open small areas of latex with a tweezer, tint the skin inside, and fill with hair gel to give the appearance of open blisters.

C. For the effect of a very old wrinkled person, apply latex and tissue to the entire face, doing one large area at a time. For a more natural wrinkled effect and finer lines (better for closeups) use the latex for wrinkling but omit the tissue.

Chapter 17

Fantasy Make-up

Fantasy make-up or 'Bal Masque' make-up as it is called in Europe, appears to have originated in the court of Marie Antoinette, in 18th Century France. One of the most popular pastimes of royalty and the wealthy was to attend grand costume parties. Elaborate masks were created by the dressmakers to coordinate with the gowns and costumes—masks that sometimes were so ornate and heavy that they had to be carried by hand and held against the face. It is said that the personal hairdresser of Marie Antoinette originated the idea of painting the mask directly onto the face with cosmetics and then glueing on precious gems, feathers or flowers to enhance the design. One could just imagine the jealousy this may have engendered among the dressmakers of the royal court.

There are times when the contemporary make-up artist may be called upon to create a make-up which is imaginative and innovative and in the Bal Masque tradition. It might be for a client who is going to a costume party or for a stage production of *Alice in Wonderland*. It may be a design for a record album cover or a special television commercial. At the very least, it would allow your artistic imagination to soar to create the ultimate in beauty fantasy.

HOW TO START

Inspiration for the facial design can come from many sources. It might be directly related to the costume such as in the case of a catlike costume calling for a feline type of make-up design. Alternatively, the material of the dress or costume may contain a form of design that can be repeated on the face, as part of the mask, such as a flower or geometric pattern. Other sources of inspiration could be found at art supply stores. There are many inexpensive books available that contain designs for flowers, birds, butterflies, and even abstracts from which you might obtain many wonderful ideas for the masks.

THE NEXT STEP

Once you have decided on the design, it should be sketched onto paper. Using the outline of a face, design the mask around the eye area. Although any part of the face may be involved in the design, the most attractive facial masks give the impression of an actual mask, often emphasizing the beauty and unique quality of the eyes. If you wish to be the most exacting, the design may be filled in with color using the actual cosmetics. One could also glue on rhinestones, flowers or feathers to the design if they are to be used in the fantasy mask. In most cases, however, a simple sketch will suffice. At this point, if it does not look good on paper it will not be attractive on the face either.

FANTASY PRODUCTS AND THEIR USE

For the basic design, you should use regular cosmetics such as eye-liner and brow pencils, eye-crayons, eye-shadows and frosted eye-powders. Theatrical lining colors are fine but be aware that generally, red colors are not to be used on the eyelid. All strong reds including lipsticks will leave a hard to remove stain on the face and eye area. It is important to start the make-up with a very heavy application of make-up base that has been well powdered. Glitter, available at the trimmings counter of most variety stores, will cling to any oily product such as colorless lip gloss. Sequins, rhinestones, artificial flowers and feathers may be glued to the skin with eyelash adhesive or spirit gum. Spirit gum may be applied to the eyebrows but it is not to be used near the eyes. When applying anything near the eyes the lash adhesive is the safest to use.

CREATING THE FANTASY MASK

As an illustration of fantasy make-up we chose to do a flower pattern design. Copying the outline of a silk flower, the design was first traced onto paper to see how it would look. Shades of yellow and blue were decided upon for the flower and green for the stem and leaves. Cosmetics in the proper shades included eye-shadows, crayons, frosted powders, glitter and eyelash adhesive.

Photo 1

Our model, Jackie, has been prepared with a basic make-up. It is important to powder down the skin to a matte finish. Basic eye make-up, some contouring, cheek color and even false lashes may be applied before the design is started.

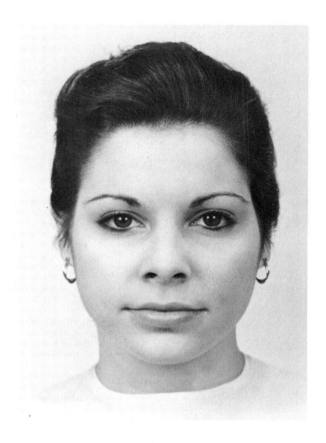

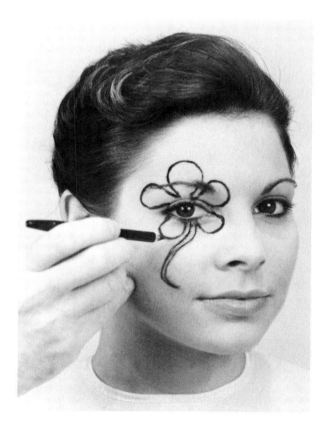

Photo 2

The design is sketched with a brow pencil directly onto the skin. One may make allowances for some change in design when transferring it to the face due to contour of the facial structure.

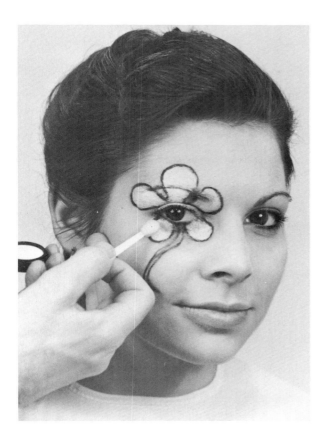

Photo 3
The flower design is filled in with yellow eye-shadow using a sponge-tipped applicator.

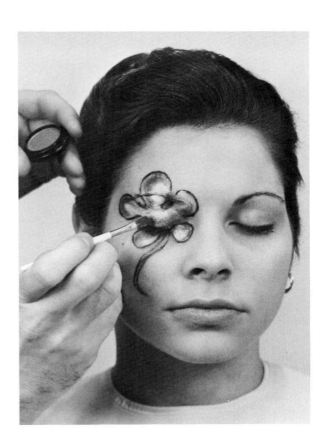

Photo 4
A teal blue eye-shadow is applied with a brush adding color and contouring to the flower petals.

Photo 5
A creamy cosmetic product is used to fill in the stem. Glitter will be pressed onto the stem area and it will cling to anything that is creamy or oily. (Do not use any form of glue for attaching glitter). The cosmetic we used was a cover-up cream which stays creamy.

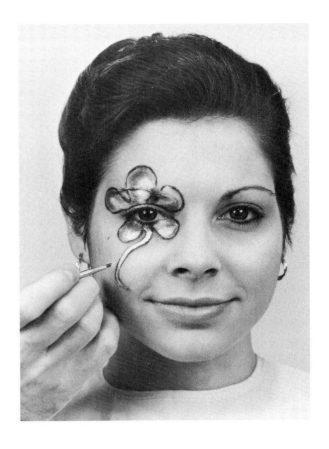

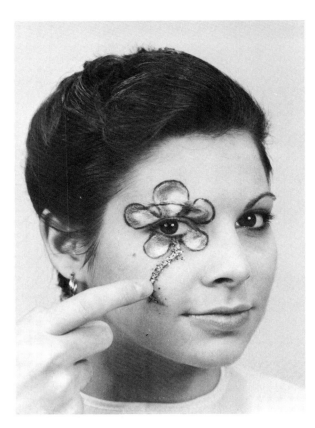

Photo 6
Multi-color glitter is pressed onto the stem design.

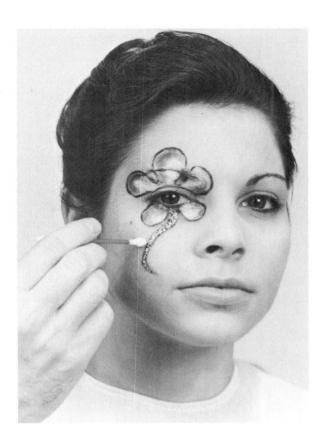

Photo 7
Glitter that fell outside of the design is brushed off with a dry cotton swab. The fact that the skin was well powdered makes this easy to do.

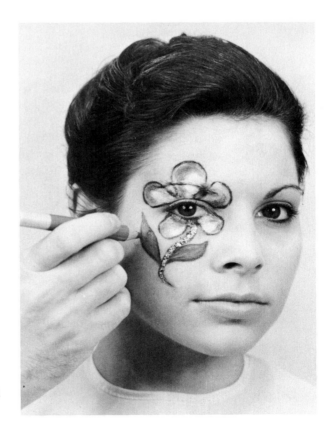

Photo 8
Leaves are sketched on and filled in with a green eye crayon.

Photo 9
A green-gold frosted powder is used to highlight
the leaves.

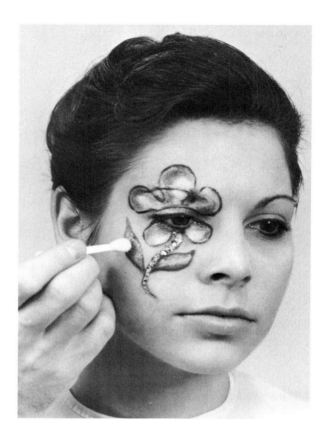

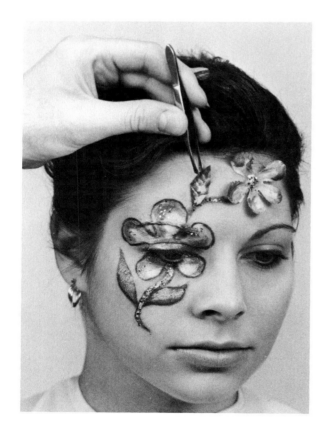

Photo 10
The original silk flower that we copied the
design from is seen being attached to the skin.
First the flower and leaf was separated from its
original stem. A stem was painted on, covered
with glitter and then the silk flower and the leaf
were glued on with eyelash adhesive.

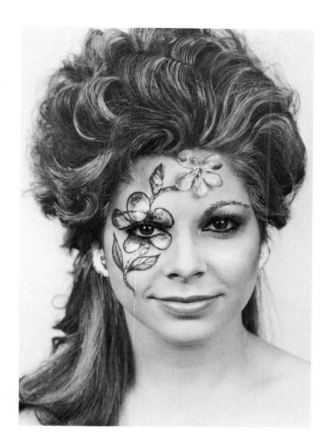

Photo 11

With a pompadour that would have gladdened the heart of Marie Antoinette herself, Jackie is certainly ready to appear at a royal ball. Her hair has been sprayed with a frosted color spray to give it highlight and color. These sprays are available wherever hair coloring products are sold and are easy to wash or brush out.

Here are a few other examples of the exotic fantasy face.

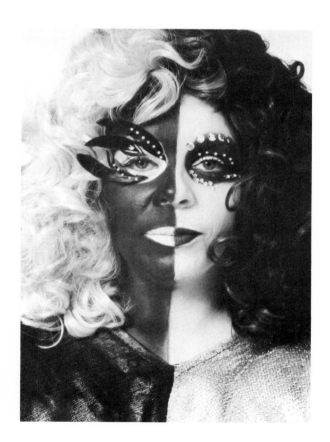

Photo 12

This two faced creation utilized black and white cake make-up, small black feathers, tiny pearls and rhinestones. The headpiece was made by cutting in half two inexpensive wigs and sewing two halves together.

Photo 13

An exotic mask is created very simply. The entire face is whitened with white cream make-up and powdered well with translucent face powder. Black eye-liner creates the eye effect and the look is completed with deep red lipstick — the only touch of color on the face.

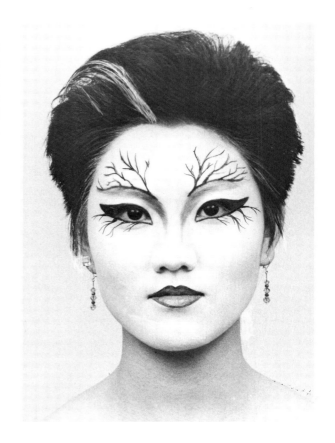

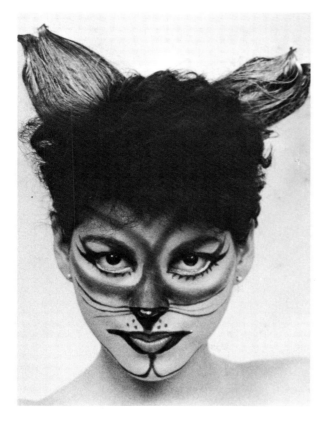

Photo 14

The background of this feline make-up is amber toned and shades of taupe and brown eye-shadow and eye-liner were used to design this cat-like fantasy. Crown hair was combed and teased up into two points to simulate ears and sprayed with blond color hair spray.

Index